Nursing Knowledge and
Theory Innovation

Pamela G. Reed, PhD, RN, FAAN, is a metatheoretician and professor at The University of Arizona College of Nursing. She also served as associate dean for academic affairs from 1995 to 2002. She was educated as a clinical nurse specialist with a focus on psychiatric-mental health nursing across the lifespan. She teaches doctoral courses on nursing metatheory, philosophy of nursing science, and theory development and evaluation. Her research has focused on spirituality, well-being and mental health at end-of-life, and on nursing philosophy and the development of nursing knowledge. She has conducted more than 14 funded research projects and 8 training grants and has received various honors for her research, including an ANF Scholars Award and the DHHS HRSA New Investigator Nursing Research Award. Her research currently focuses on end-of-life family caregiver well-being and spiritual and scientific ways of knowing.

Dr. Reed has developed a nursing theory of self-transcendence used by researchers around the world. She has also produced two widely used research instruments, the *Spiritual Perspective Scale* and the *Self-Transcendence Scale*, and consults nationally on spirituality-related measurement and research. She has received eight awards for outstanding teaching and has been visiting scholar at New York University and Duke University Center for Spirituality, Theology and Health, among other universities. She was a contributing editor to *Nursing Science Quarterly* and, along with Dr. Nelma Shearer, edits the theory textbook *Perspectives on Nursing Theory* for doctoral education. She has presented more than 40 invited papers, including most recently several national papers on the practice of nursing science and on nursing knowledge production through theory and inquiry in practice. She has published more than 23 book chapters and more than 70 peer-reviewed articles. She is a member of Sigma Theta Tau International and is a fellow in the American Academy of Nursing. She resides with her family in Tucson, Arizona.

Nelma B. Crawford Shearer, PhD, RN, is a researcher, associate professor and codirector of the Hartford Center of Geriatric Nursing Excellence at Arizona State University College of Nursing and Health Innovation. Her teaching responsibilities focus on theoretical foundations of nursing at the graduate and doctoral level, including a course on theoretical foundations of doctoral education for advanced nursing practice. She is an American Nurses Foundation scholar and a John A. Hartford Foundation Institute of Geriatric Nursing Research scholar. In 2006, she received the Geriatric Nursing Research award from the Western Institute of Nursing in partnership with the Hartford Institute for Geriatric Nursing.

Dr. Shearer conducts research into the process of promoting health empowerment in older adults with the goal of optimizing their well-being. She has received funding from the National Institute of Nursing Research to test her theory-based health empowerment intervention with homebound older adults. In addition, she, as a coinvestigator with an ASU colleague, has received funding for research projects including the Hartford Foundation for Building Academic Geriatric Nursing Capacity in Arizona and the Southwest and funding for program grants through the HRSA Comprehensive Geriatric Education Program. She has published 15 peer-reviewed journal articles and several book chapters and, with Dr. Reed, edits the textbook *Perspectives on Nursing Theory*. She has delivered more than 25 scholarly presentations, many of which focus on the development and testing of her theory-based empowerment intervention. She is currently vice president of the Society of Rogerian Scholars International Organization and a member of Sigma Theta Tau International and the Western Institute of Nursing Research. She resides with her family in Tempe, Arizona.

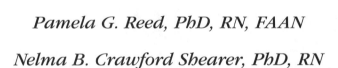

Nursing Knowledge and Theory Innovation

Advancing the Science of Practice

Pamela G. Reed, PhD, RN, FAAN

Nelma B. Crawford Shearer, PhD, RN

SPRINGER PUBLISHING COMPANY

NEW YORK

Springer Publishing Company, LLC
11 West 42nd Street
New York, NY 10036
www.springerpub.com

Acquisitions Editor: Margaret Zuccarini
Project Manager: Ashita Shah, Newgen Imaging
Composition: Newgen Imaging

ISBN: 978-0-8261-1892-9
E-book ISBN: 978-0-8261-1893-6

11 12 13 14   5 4 3 2 1

The author and the publisher of this Work have made every effort to use sources believed to be reliable to provide information that is accurate and compatible with the standards generally accepted at the time of publication. Because medical science is continually advancing, our knowledge base continues to expand. Therefore, as new information becomes available, changes in procedures become necessary. We recommend that the reader always consult current research and specific institutional policies before performing any clinical procedure. The author and publisher shall not be liable for any special, consequential, or exemplary damages resulting, in whole or in part, from the readers' use of, or reliance on, the information contained in this book. The publisher has no responsibility for the persistence or accuracy of URLs for external or third-party Internet Web sites referred to in this publication and does not guarantee that any content on such Web sites is, or will remain, accurate or appropriate.

Library of Congress Cataloging-in-Publication Data
Reed, Pamela G., 1952–
    Nursing knowledge and theory innovation : advancing the science of practice /
Pamela G. Reed, Nelma B.C. Shearer.
       p. ; cm.
    Includes bibliographical references and index.
    ISBN 978-0-8261-1892-9 — ISBN 978-0-8261-1893-6 (E-book)
    1. Nursing—Research. 2. Nursing—Practice. 3. Nursing—Philosophy.
4. Knowledge and learning. I. Shearer, Nelma B. Crawford, 1950– II. Title.
    [DNLM: 1. Nursing Theory. 2. Health Knowledge, Attitudes, Practice.
3. Nurse's Practice Patterns. WY 86]
    RT81.5.R44 2011
    610.73—dc22   2010051480

Special discounts on bulk quantities of our books are available to corporations, professional associations, pharmaceutical companies, health care organizations, and other qualifying groups.

If you are interested in a custom book, including chapters from more than one of our titles, we can provide that service as well.

For details, please contact:
Special Sales Department, Springer Publishing Company, LLC
11 West 42nd Street, 15th Floor, New York, NY 10036–8002
Phone: 877–687–7476 or 212–431–4370; Fax: 212–941–7842
Email: sales@springerpub.com

Printed in the United States of America by Hamilton Printing

*We dedicate this book to our students and colleagues
who share our interest in the synergy within
the science and practice of nursing.*

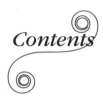

Contents

Contributors

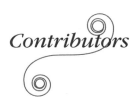

Catherine Johnson, PhD, PNP, FNP
Associate Professor, Mt. Carmel College of Nursing, Columbus, Ohio

Elaine G. Jones, PhD, RN, FAANP
Associate Professor, Director of Honors Program, The University of Arizona, College of Nursing, Tucson, Arizona

Lisa A. Lawrence, PhD, RN
Assistant Professor, Northern Michigan University, School of Nursing, Marquette, Michigan

Donna Behler McArthur, PhD, FNP-BC, FAANP
Professor, Director, DNP Program, Vanderbilt University, School of Nursing, Nashville, Tennessee

Cathleen Michaels, PhD, RN, FNAP, FAAN
Clinical Associate Professor, The University of Arizona, College of Nursing, Tucson, Arizona

Pamela G. Reed, PhD, RN, FAAN
Professor, The University of Arizona, College of Nursing, Tucson, Arizona

Gary Rolfe, PhD, MA, BSc, RMN, PGCEA
Professor of Nursing, School of Health Science, Swansea University, Swansea, Wales

Nelma B. Crawford Shearer, PhD, RN
Associate Professor and Co-Director, Hartford Center of Geriatric Nursing Excellence, Arizona State University, College of Nursing & Health Innovation, Phoenix, Arizona

Donna M. Velasquez, PhD, RN, FNP-BC, FAANP
Clinical Associate Professor, FNP DNP Coordinator, Arizona State University, College of Nursing & Health Innovation, Phoenix, Arizona

Foreword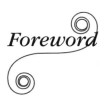

This book, as stated by the editors in their preface, is intended to highlight the need to consider knowledge development in nursing in the context of practice and to show ways for advanced nursing clinicians to participate in knowledge development. This intention and the offerings in the chapters emphasize the nature of nursing knowledge characterized as "human practice science" (Kim, 2010). Nursing's knowledge system as a human practice science is concerned with developing knowledge for practice; the knowledge that is relevant to and needed in practice. As a human practice science, nursing has to address epistemic questions regarding specific human conditions within the nursing domains and those related to how to improve such human conditions from the nursing perspective. As stated by Rolfe in Chapter 4, the ultimate goal of nursing inquiry is to develop practice rather than simply to develop theory. This suggests a differentiation between the basic sciences and the applied sciences of which human practice sciences are examples in terms of both the aims of knowledge development and the sorts of knowledge to be developed in scientific disciplines. Epistemic questions for the basic sciences rest with humans' fundamental search for understanding and explanations about the nature, whereas those for the applied sciences rest with human's search for improving human lot and for correcting various inadequacies that occur in the nature.

Nursing as a knowledge system thus aims for gaining knowledge that can shape nursing practice to be consequential in influencing human's healthful living. To develop knowledge that is intentionally relevant to nursing practice, it is necessary for the process of knowledge development to be embedded in nursing practice.

Unfortunately, the development of nursing knowledge during the past several decades has followed the course that has been mapped out and followed by various scientific fields within which the objectification of subject matters is the primary mode of scientific work. This, along with other social forces, has led to the separation of theorists/scholars/researchers/academicians from practitioners and has created a great chasm between theory and practice in nursing. Although such compartmentalization does not necessarily mean that the knowledge that has been developed and is being developed in nursing is not addressing important questions in nursing practice, there has been a great deal of anxiety regarding the significance of this objectified, generalized knowledge for influencing practice. The recent institutionalization of an educational route for advanced expert clinicians through the practice-focused doctoral preparation in nursing (DNP) has stimulated a rethinking regarding this bifurcation between theory and practice, between researcher and practitioner, and between generalized knowledge and situated knowledge. It has been advocated that advanced expert clinicians prepared in such doctoral programs have to assume the role of bridging knowledge development with knowledge use in practice as well as to take up the pivotal position through which practice-relevant epistemic questions are raised and addressed for knowledge development. There are many models for the engagement of advanced expert clinicians in nursing knowledge development. Several models are presented in this book.

A major model is presented in Chapter 1 by Reed in which the practice-based knowledge development in nursing is viewed to require an integration of the practice of science and the practice of nursing within the six turns of the spiral path of knowledge development. In this model, shaping of clinicians' engagement in nursing knowledge development is viewed to be accomplished by one's positions and sensitivity in addressing knowledge development questions in practice. Another model advocated in Chapter 2 by Velasquez, McArthur, and Johnson suggests the practitioner-theorist-researcher role for clinicians in nursing knowledge development as contrast to the scientist-theorist-researcher role for academics, applying exploration, explication, engagement, and optimization as the major processes for practice-based knowledge generation. On the other hand, Rolfe in Chapter 4 recommends a specific epistemology of nursing as a reflexive science in which practice and research are integrated in producing "a science of the unique." For Rolfe, the engagement of a practitioner in *praxis* is necessarily a knowledge-generating occasion in which an integration of theory, research, and practice occurs through reflection, reflexivity, and on-the-spot experimentation. Theory development by practitioners is proposed through the application of nontraditional modes of theoretical thinking unique to practice situations especially for formalizing personal theories and identifying key areas of inquiry arising from practice in Chapter 7 by Reed. Jones in Chapter 8 also suggests clinical scholarship for engagement in translational research and revisional theory development as one approach.

From the perspective culminating from the proposals made in this book and the current epistemic culture of nursing as a scientific discipline, we can raise three questions:

1. Is there a specific and different role to be played by advanced clinicians in nursing knowledge development, adopting unique approaches that are embedded in practice? If so, what is the contribution by such efforts on the whole schema of nursing knowledge development?
2. Does nursing have to identify its discipline-specific methods for knowledge development to address the unique features of nursing practice and nursing's epistemic concerns?
3. What would be required of advanced clinicians to advocate for and participate in the role in nursing knowledge development?

The first question is addressed by several authors in this book. Practice occurs in a specific clinical site that is unique and nonrepeating and in which clinicians are engaged in clinical actions both with clients and for clients. Clinicians have to meld together the knowledge, skills, intuitions, experiences, understandings, and self to bring about accountability to one's practice. Knowledge-based practice that goes beyond evidence-based practice is required at the base guided by the assumptions that (a) the knowledge for nursing practice refers to a body of specialized knowledge that is multidimensional, complex in its configuration, and derived from multiple sources, (b) the processes by which individual practitioners use and develop knowledge in practice are context-specific, situated, and individualistic in the sense that each practice instance is unique in its presentation of a client's conditions, problems, trajectory, history, and context, and (c) the practitioner is the user, synthesizer, and generator of knowledge who must adopt certain attitudinal, cognitive, strategic, and action processes (Kim, 2006). This is a similar notion as the concept of theory-based practice mentioned by Reed in Chapter 12. It requires practitioners to apply creative, analytic, and dialogical methods to synthesize knowledge and experience to fit into specific clinical situations so that the knowledge-based practice becomes exemplary. In addition, such exemplary practice occasions are exactly the sites from which practice-based knowledge development can occur as demonstrated by Reed in Chapter 12. In practice-based knowledge development, identification of various practice models "created" in specific clinical situations can lead to the development of theories for practice and formalization of knowledge synthesis; respecifications of general theories addressing specific clinical and contextual requirements may emerge as revisions of theories; or testing of situation-specific theories (Im & Meleis, 1999) in practice may result in clinical validation or modification. Practice-based knowledge developed by such modes thus can bridge the generalized knowledge to practice.

The second question is taken up by Rolfe in Chapter 4 as well as in his earlier work (Rolfe, 2006), and by other authors in the literature, notably by Gadow for local narratives (1995) and Newman for research as praxis (1997). In this stance, nursing knowledge is viewed to be embedded in practice of specific, existential frames from which knowledge both emerges and is formalized. Nursing knowledge from this perspective is local, unique, and situated and is generated as informal theories, local narratives, and praxis itself. Practitioners in practice are at the center of knowledge development as engagers in praxis that integrates research into practice.

The third question is a critical question for the preparation of advanced expert clinicians, as the question assumes that such practitioners are not simply users of knowledge but are knowledge generators as well. Such practitioners need to develop an attitude and methods for an active role in knowledge development. Johnson and Reed advocate mindfulness practice in Chapter 5 as a way for practitioners to stay tuned to one's own practice, acknowledging knowledge integration and knowledge creation in practice. Schön in his work on reflective practice (1983) proposes ways for practitioners to be open and critical of one's practice through reflection-in-action and reflection-on-action, which can be used as methods for discovering knowing in practice. Similarly, Argyris, Putnam, and Smith (1985) advanced action science as a method for practitioners to engage in the Model II learning and engage in an ongoing examination of one's own practice for knowledge generation. Critical reflective inquiry suggests one approach by which practitioners can assume a self-critiquing stance regarding one's practice and engage in developing knowledge from practice (Kim, 1999). The concept of scientist-practitioner advanced for clinical psychologists from the Boulder Agenda of the 1940s is still viable as a model to incorporate the researcher role with the practice role for clinicians. Advanced expert clinicians need to become competent in applying research methods that are specifically appropriate for the practitioner-scientist role, such as case-study methods, action research, fieldwork methods, quasi experiments, and narrative analysis as well as various theory revision approaches applicable in one's own practice, some of which are presented in this book.

This book, departing from offering the traditional theory-development approaches, points to the areas that need to be deeply investigated by students in DNP programs, practicing expert clinicians, and clinical nursing researchers to be both inculcated into the role of clinician in nursing knowledge development and introduced to various extant and noble approaches appropriate for practice-based knowledge development.

Hesook Suzie Kim, PhD, RN

References

Argyris, C., Putnam, R., & Smith, D. (1985). *Action science.* San Francisco: Jossey-Bass.

Gadow, S. (1995). Narrative and exploration: Toward a poetics of knowledge in nursing. *Nursing Inquiry, 2,* 211–214.

Im, E. O., & Meleis, A. I. (1999). Situation-specific theories: Philosophical roots, properties, and approach. *Advances in Nursing Science, 22,* 11–24.

Kim, H. S. (1999). Critical reflective inquiry for knowledge development in nursing practice. *Journal of Advanced Nursing, 29,* 1205–1212.

Kim, H. S. (2006). Knowledge synthesis and use in practice—Debunking "evidence-based." *Klinisk sygepleje, 20*(2), 24–34.

Kim, H. S. (2010). *The nature of theoretical thinking in nursing* (3rd ed.). New York: Springer.

Newman, M. A. (1997). Experiencing the whole: Health as expanding consciousness: State of the art. *Advances in Nursing Science, 20,* 34–39.

Rolfe, G. (2006). Nursing praxis and the science of the unique. *Nursing Science Quarterly, 19,* 39–43.

Schön, D. (1983). *The reflective practitioner.* New York: Basic Books.

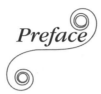

Preface

How does nursing knowledge come into being? This is not a new question nor can it be answered simply by referring to the scientific method or evidence-based practice. The current shift in nursing toward educating many more doctoral-level practitioners compels us to revisit this question from a 21st-century perspective. Science, philosophy, theory, and practice exist in a complex relationship that generates knowledge for nursing. However, the knowledge-generating capacity of the context of practice and practicing nurses has not been fully recognized. The burgeoning of graduate-level practicing nurses presents new opportunities for building nursing knowledge to meet society's health care needs. In addition, emphasizing the practice lens in nursing's network of knowledge enriches the theory base for addressing nursing problems.

Focus of the Book

The focus of this book is nursing knowledge and theory development in practice. A doctoral-level nurse, whether PhD or DNP prepared, is expected to both *use* and *develop* knowledge (Dracup, Cronenwett, Meleis, Benner, 2005, p. 179). In terms of knowledge development, it is generally thought that researchers and theorists provide the new knowledge and theories for the practicing nurses to apply, evaluate, and perhaps modify in their practice. New knowledge, whether from published evidence or existing theories, flows primarily from outside the context of the nurse's practice. Practicing nurses also look within practice for knowledge, for example, in terms of their immediate observations, interactions with patients and families, conversations with colleagues, and expert judgment. However, what goes unrecognized in health care and unclaimed by nurses is the theoretical thinking that occurs in this process and nurses' capacity to develop theory *for* practice *in* practice. Theoretical thinking allows problems and their explanations to emerge in practice with patients and families, rather than to exist as predescribed problems and prescribed solutions.

The innovation in knowledge development proposed in this book is intended to inspire and support nurses' theoretical thinking in practice and expand our repertoire of strategies for theory development. Few writings in nursing have addressed how nursing knowledge comes into being in practice; instead, theory texts have addressed creative applications of theory to practice and testing theory in research. The literature is dominated by a focus on *application*, not *origination*, of knowledge in practice because, in part, scientific knowledge traditionally has been developed out of the contexts in which it is used and is not directly applicable to practice. In addition, the concern over the *amount* of knowledge developed is being replaced with concerns about *how* knowledge is developed amid the proliferation of research findings and other evidence for practice (Stehr, 2004). Thus, a frontier in knowledge development is the production of nursing knowledge and theory in the patient-centered context of nursing practice.

A Call for Transformation

The perspectives on knowledge development in this book support the four key recommendations for educating nurses outlined by Benner, Sutphen, Leonar, and Day (2009) in their call for radical transformation of nursing programs. That is, this book encourages development of contextualized knowledge for practice; promotes more deliberate strategies to link theory to practice; supports the emphasis on clinical imagination in exploring new ways of reasoning and theorizing in practice beyond the focus on critical thinking; and supports the transformation of practicing nurses' identity by encouraging and guiding their participation as knowledge producers beyond that of knowledge users in practice. Innovative theoretical thinking in practice and the various knowledge sources from which it draws must not be eclipsed by any of the more familiar reasoning processes of critical thinking, problem solving, or decision making (Lester & Piore, 2004).

Intended Audience of the Book

This textbook is intended for a graduate-level nursing students, particularly students enrolled in Doctor of Nursing Practice (DNP) programs. The book is also intended for PhD nursing students, as they increasingly are bringing to their research a practice-centered focus. It will also be useful for nurse practitioner students or master's-level nursing students enrolled in a theory course or planning their master's research project. Doctorally prepared nurses and faculty will also find this book relevant in their scholarly work.

Structure of the Book

This book presents a new philosophic stance and historical, practical, and theoretical perspectives regarding practice-based theory and knowledge development. Five chapters were developed as *Interludes* where readers can pause and explore specific aspects of knowledge development in reference to their own nursing practice and research.

The Spiral Path. Chapter 1 presents a model of the geography of nursing knowledge and how theory evolves, with emphasis on theoretical thinking in practice. The model is presented in the form of a *spiral path* that integrates six elements in knowledge development: philosophy of nursing, philosophy of science, practice of science, practice of nursing, theoretical thinking, and theory. The model is open to modification. A new philosophic perspective, called *intermodernism*, is discussed in reference to each element of nursing knowledge in the spiral path. Intermodernism is a philosophy of science that sits between modernism and postmodernism.

The subsequent chapters are stops along the path to address special areas with an emphasis on practice in nursing knowledge. Interlude chapters focus on strategies and perspectives that facilitate knowledge development and theoretical thinking in practice. The chapters are written from each author's first-hand experience in a particular dimension of knowledge development.

Chapter 2 squarely addresses the roles of PhD and DNP nurses in knowledge development, and the authors propose a conceptual model, outlining how each role contributes in unique and shared ways to the development of nursing knowledge. Chapters 3, 5, 7, 9, and 11 are interludes designed to present a specific approach that fosters theoretical thinking and theory development. These approaches range from *creating a Mandala* to clarify one's philosophy of nursing and *practicing mindfulness* to sensitize one to theoretical concepts embedded in practice, to a *community-based praxis* approach in theory development and specific *steps in reformulating* a practice-based nursing concept. Two other chapters discuss philosophical and practical dimensions of practice-based theory development. An additional chapter provides a historical perspective and future projections on clinical scholarship in nursing.

The chapters in this book will help students to (a) become aware of their own philosophical and theoretical ideas and knowledge embedded in their practice and (b) learn strategies for developing theory-based knowledge—strategies that are practice relevant and practice based. The book balances theoretical and philosophical ideas with the practical. In addition, it includes examples of concrete strategies that can be used by nurses in their work with individuals, groups, and communities. Although the chapters elaborate on various aspects of knowledge development, they neither exhaust the possibilities nor bring closure to how nursing knowledge comes into being. This remains very much an open topic that requires continued inquiry and dialogue.

Summary

This book is unique in its contribution to the theory textbook literature with its focus on expanding nursing's knowledge-building capacity by engaging practicing nurses in theory and knowledge development. Scholars within and outside of nursing are calling for a more active role of practitioners in developing new knowledge for a discipline. Moreover, nurses themselves increasingly recognize the importance of theoretical knowledge in understanding and communicating the complex problems that confront them in their practice.

In sharing the ideas in this book, we seek to inspire and equip nursing students with the tools to make theory more relevant to their own practice, to become aware of and develop their own theoretical ideas in practice, and in doing this advance practice while building creativity and confidence in their own knowledge. Recognition of the theoretical thinking that occurs within evidence-based practice invites continued dialogue concerning how we think about nurses' scholarly practice and educate nurses at graduate and doctoral levels.

References

Benner, P., Sutphen, M., Leonard, V., & Day, L. (2010). *Educating nurses: A call for radical transformation.* Stanford, CA: The Carnegie Foundations for the Advancement of Teaching.

Dracup, K., Cronenwett, L., Meleis, A. I., & Benner, P. (2005). Reflections on the doctorate of nursing practice. *Nursing Outlook, 53*, 177–182.

Lester, R. K., & Piore, M. J. (2004). *Innovation—The missing dimension.* Cambridge, MA: Harvard University Press.

Stehr, N. (Ed.). (2004). *The governance of knowledge.* New Brunswick, NJ: Transaction.

Acknowledgments

Many people have contributed to making this book a success for nursing. We first thank the contributors whose timeless ideas and insights about nursing are recorded between the covers of this book. Their chapters comprise the substance of the book, and together, provide the practice lens for exploring new thinking about knowledge development in nursing.

We thank our students—past, present, and future—who helped inspire the creation of this book. It is our hope that the chapters will further students' learning and equip them with the tools to make theory more relevant to their own practice, to develop their own theoretical ideas in practice, and in so doing advance practice while building nursing knowledge. Special acknowledgment goes to Kathryn Bevacqua, Media Specialist, University of Arizona College of Nursing, whose creative work on the models for the Chapters 1 and 2 figures and the book cover is pure evidence of knowledge production through expert artistic practice.

We appreciate everyone at Springer Publishing Company for their careful, expert work in transforming ideas about theory innovation and knowledge development in nursing practice and science into this portable package. We especially thank Margaret Zuccarini, executive acquisitions editor at Springer Publishing Company, for her meticulous guidance throughout the project and particularly for listening to our idea and then championing the book to the editorial board. We also acknowledge Christina Ferraro, assistant editor, and Elizabeth Stump, former assistant editor at Springer Publishing Company, for their abiding attention to detail in pulling everything together.

The Spiral Path of Nursing Knowledge

Pamela G. Reed

How does that which we call nursing knowledge come into being?

In the late 19th century, Britain's Florence Nightingale professionalized nursing practice by enacting her theoretical ideas about the significance of the physical and social environment in human health and well-being. Nightingale's focus on facilitating the person's inner processes of healing by tending to the environment, along with her expertise in statistics and other ways of knowing, made her a compelling leader for nursing science and practice. As the 20th century progressed, new leaders in theoretical thinking energized nursing's advancement in education, research, and practice. Hildegard Peplau's (1952) theory of interpersonal relations introduced a major scientific treatise on the nurse–patient relationship, which remains a defining focus of nursing practice. Martha Rogers' (1970) work on the theoretical basis of nursing presented progressive ideas about human complexity and person–environment processes that are still unfolding today in contemporary theorizing and science. Many other notable theorists—including some of you—have joined and will join these three historical icons to advance the role of nursing in the knowledge and practice of health care.

Nursing has a rich history of theoretical thinkers. Nursing scientist scholars who were first educated in theory-based or theory-enriched disciplines like sociology, psychology, anthropology, and education provided an abundance of theoretical thinking and conceptual systems of, and for, nursing. Nurses educated in graduate-level nursing programs followed and produced theories and theory-related writings about nursing. Because of this, we may take for granted what some fields (e.g., McQueen, 2007) still quest for—a theoretical basis for the profession.

The purpose of this chapter is to provide an overview of a path of nursing knowledge that encourages new or renewed participation among nurses, particularly practicing nurses, in developing knowledge for the discipline. It is a path *of,* rather than *to,* knowledge because there is no ultimate goal or final theory in knowledge development. The theories of today need to be sensitive to the given situation and changing problems and experiences, yet also illuminate patterns that broaden understanding of nursing phenomena. The path offers up a tentative yet useful form of knowledge called "theories," but invariably spirals us forward through the process of knowledge building.

The linchpin of this path is the practice of nursing, that is, the practice of *facilitating processes of health and well-being within and among human systems across a diversity of environments*. The integral link between practice and knowledge is not new, and emphasizing this link in nursing's network of knowledge presents some challenges for science and theory development. However, the challenges are worthwhile given their potential for furthering nursing's unique and innovative contributions to human health and health care. This chapter is a beginning in what I hope will become an extended dialogue about innovations in developing nursing knowledge. Authors of subsequent chapters take up the dialogue from their various practices and perspectives.

THE SPIRAL PATH

Along the hiking trails in mountains where the ancients once walked, you can spot petroglyphs, ancient carvings or inscriptions, embedded in the rocks and boulders. Some of these depict a spiral form, which is found on every continent. I used this spiral form to symbolize a process of knowledge development in nursing (see Figure 1.1). To the ancient people, the spiral form represented one of various ideas that can apply to the process of knowledge development: an energy; a life-giving source like water; a process of emerging or transcending; a portal or gateway from the mundane to the eternal realms; or perhaps most relevant to the career of being a nursing student or scholar is its symbolization of a life journey and the challenges for growth faced along the way.

The petroglyph that inspired the spiral design resembles a foot path, earthy and imperfect, of various turns. It is not a perfect spiral like the artificial depiction you might find in a catalog, but rather, it is imperfect to represent the natural, dynamic, and often messy processes of nursing practice, science, and theorizing.

The spiral path has six turns—there could be more or fewer. Each turn corresponds to a particular focus and tool of inquiry for knowledge development. The components of the Path are not arranged hierarchically, unlike other models of the structure of nursing knowledge. Instead, the spiral is an ongoing and nonlinear path, open to influences that can be incorporated for innovative and unpredictable change. The Path, rather than being a series of concentric circles, is a spiral form to convey continuity across the dimensions; from everyday knowledge work to scientific theories, knowledge construction is a "fundamentally continuous" process, as described by the practicing scientist Fleck in his book on comparative epistemology, *Genesis and development of a science fact* (cited in Smith, 2005, p. 26).

The spiral path is a way of thinking about how various components of knowledge development are organized and related. What are listed here may be modified or expanded, depending on your context of nursing science and practice, and depending upon what you would like to emphasize—a pragmatic turn? an ethical

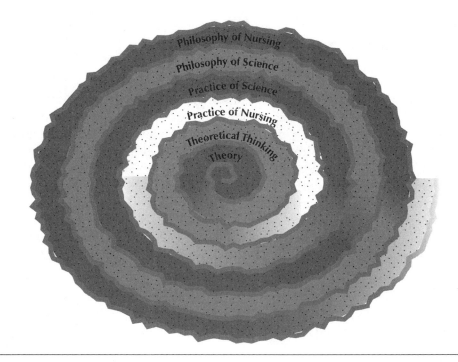

FIGURE 1.1

The Spiral Path of Nursing Knowledge.

turn? or a spiritual turn? It is likely, though, that any approach to knowledge development involves a dynamic network or web of components that includes philosophical, empirical, and theoretical dimensions of the discipline.

Knowledge development is, above all, an emergent process, paralleling the process of change that its creators undergo over time—open and ongoing, developmental and sometimes decremental, patterned yet unpredictable, complex yet organized, bringing forth outcomes that are greater than the sum of its various turns, but still influenced by each turn. The scientific knowledge produced, as indicated by the *theory* circle, is not necessarily cumulative nor is it unchanging or unchangeable, but it is relevant to the practice situation or problems to which it is linked. And of course, other forms of knowledge inhabit the Path. Nursing knowledge is enriched by many patterns of knowing, which inform, and are informed by, the scientific pattern represented by the theory component of the Path.

THE CONTEXT OF THEORY

Theory is a central component in the path of nursing knowledge. Theory is the "vehicle of scientific knowledge, and one way or another become[s] involved in most aspects of the scientific enterprise" (Suppe, 1977, p. 3). Theory exists within a context of philosophical, empirical, and theoretical dimensions, and has a path of inquiry whereby theory emerges out of nursing practice and research. Theory also functions reflexively to inform nurses' practice and research. This path of inquiry is represented in Figure 1.1, which highlights key aspects of the philosophical, empirical, and theoretical dimensions of knowledge development.

Philosophical Dimension

The philosophical dimension consists of conceptual components that influence knowledge development, including philosophy of science, the nursing metaparadigm, and philosophy of nursing as well as personal beliefs and values. These philosophical components express the conceptual perspectives that influence (or at least are related to) the *substantive* focus of theories (ontology) and the *process* focus on empirical methods and patterns of knowing and warranting knowledge (epistemology) in a discipline. The philosophical dimension broadly describes the way things are from a certain perspective of reality, and the way things should be from a certain perspective of morality. In Figure 1.1 of the Path, these dimensions are represented by the *Philosophy of Nursing* and the *Philosophy of Science*.

Empirical Dimension

The empirical components are the observables used in knowledge generation as obtained directly or indirectly through the senses, for example, through the nurse's personal life experiences, nursing practice and other professional experiences, the patient's assessed needs and perspectives, research methods of observation and measurement of variables in the theory, and empirical findings from research. Of course, because our body and mind are *not* distinct Cartesian entities, anything obtained through the senses is already interpreted, as influenced by conceptual (philosophical and theoretical) dimensions. These dimensions, represented by the *Practice of Science* and the *Practice of Nursing* in Figure 1.1, sit between the philosophical and theoretical dimensions in the Path figure because these material, embodied practices are considered to be a linchpin in nursing knowledge development.

Theoretical Dimension

The theoretical dimension in the path of knowledge involves both a process and product, that is, *theoretical thinking* and the conceptual structure called a *theory*, respectively as represented toward the center of the Path in Figure 1.1. Theories are open systems, which are amenable to change and possible improvement by critique, modification, and refinement through ongoing theory development and evaluation. Theory development is influenced by both the philosophical and empirical dimensions. Theories link the everyday world of practice and the philosophical perspectives of reality.

METATHEORY

Metatheory is a word that ties together the three areas addressed in the Path. Metatheory refers to the study of how the philosophical, theoretical, and empirical components in the structure of knowledge work together to produce nursing theory. It is a term used across disciplines, and sometimes it is used to refer to an overarching theory. But most often it is used, as described here, in the broader philosophical context of knowledge development rather than as a specific theoretical perspective. Metatheory is not a theory per se but rather a domain of conceptual tools that inform development of *substantive* theory, theoretical concepts, and research design.

Nursing metatheory identifies the domain of nursing that addresses the philosophical perspectives, substantive focuses, and methods concerning nursing knowledge. *Metatheory* encompasses all of the elements that are used in developing nursing knowledge, especially the following: philosophies and methods of science; nursing ontology and epistemology; the nursing metaparadigm and the conceptual models that elaborate on the metaparadigm concepts; middle range and other levels of theories; and the nurses' personal values and professional practice domain (Reed, 2010). These metatheoretical tools inform and influence the development of theories and theoretical concepts (Sibeon, 2007).

It is important to attend to these metatheoretical components, which are represented in the Path of Nursing Knowledge, because they account for the human context of science. While theory and knowledge development are addressed here as primarily scientific activities, nonetheless they are human activities—replete with personal values, fallibility, and biases, and influenced by historical, cultural, and social contexts. This fact, along with the inability to remove the challenges and doubts that it interjects into our quest for knowledge, is regarded amusingly by Smith (2005) as *the* scandal of philosophy of science, and it has nearly paralyzed the creativity and productivity of some philosophers and scientists! But as nurses, we embrace the human messiness of knowledge development, as we do in our nursing interactions with people in the midst of wellness and illness, living and dying. Indeed, the context of discovery is very much a part of the metatheoretical concerns about the development and justification of scientific knowledge and theories. And so, let's take a brief tour around this path of nursing knowledge, one step at a time.

PHILOSOPHY OF NURSING

The Path begins anywhere, but we will start at the outmost circle, with the turn toward our own philosophy of nursing. Scholars tell us that all knowledge begins and ends with philosophy and nurses are philosophers! Whenever you wrestle with questions about what is morally right or wrong in a patient care situation, when you reflect on what you believe relative to your choices and actions as a practitioner or a teacher or researcher, when you reflect on what you value and its influence on your science or practice, when you're faced with gray situations where there is no one right answer or approach—you are engaging in philosophical inquiry, whether or not you have been formally prepared in the logic and theory behind it.

Philosophers confront questions that cannot be answered by scientific inquiry, but philosophical inquiry nonetheless can provide a window into understanding what evidence you choose to believe in and why, what health goals you pursue in research, and what health goals and behaviors you value for yourself and your patients.

Reflexivity is an important attitude, from a stance both within and outside the situation, to consider explanations, values, and influences on your beliefs and goals in nursing. You can construct your own philosophy of science by engaging in philosophical inquiry, reflecting on and writing down the following elements: your ontological and epistemological views, your metaparadigmatic statement about nursing, and the personal values and professional and life experiences that may influence these views.

PHILOSOPHICAL INQUIRY

Philosophical inquiry is a tool in knowledge development because it raises awareness of factors that influence or inspire your knowledge development in practice and research. Questioning is a key practice within philosophical inquiry. To question is to "decline to take for granted" (Smith, 2005, p. 7). Some of the purposes of philosophical inquiry are as follows:

- To question seemingly self-evident assumptions, beliefs, values
- To expose hidden assumptions and distorted means of thinking
- To provide a context and comprehensive views of the discipline for research and practice
- To address questions that science cannot address (metaphysical, ontological, epistemological, ethical)
- To help ensure that science does not violate the values of the nursing profession
- To keep the discipline open to change through use of reason and reflection

I can learn something about your philosophy of nursing by asking you to respond to questions like the following: *What is nursing? What are the elements of a human being that nursing should attend to? Which ones are the most important? Is there an underlying order to the universe or is it mostly chaos and we make it seem orderly by our beliefs or research methods we impose on the world? Is there a Truth out there or is it found within each individual or group? How do you define health, and is it ethical to apply your definition to patients and research participants?* Philosophers dare to interrogate themselves and others with questions about disciplinary values that are not supposed to be questioned, for example, values about professionalism in nursing, the morality of promoting compliance, the inherent goodness of the nurse–patient relationship, or the scientific value in quantifying spirituality. These questions relate to one of the six areas of philosophical inquiry listed in Table 1.1.

ONTOLOGY

Ontology addresses the substance or subject matter of the discipline, and in so doing, defines what the discipline considers relevant *focuses* for knowledge development and practice. (Incidentally, epistemology addresses the *methods* of or how

TABLE 1.1

Areas of Philosophical Inquiry

1. *Metaphysics*—nature of reality, existence, and substance of the universe
   What is the nature of a realm of reality beyond the empirical universe?

2. *Ontology*—nature of being of a discipline
   What is the focus or substance of a discipline?

3. *Epistemology*—nature of knowledge and truth
   How is knowledge formed and warranted in a given discipline?

4. *Axiology*—nature of values in science
   How does the science handle values in its practice and science?

5. *Ethics*—nature of human conduct
   What morals and codes of conduct govern scientific practices in the discipline?

6. *Aesthetics*—nature of beauty
   What is considered "beauty" in nursing? Is being healthy beauty? Are the practices of nursing care expressions of beauty?

we go about building knowledge about the substance of a discipline.) The term *ontology* has been defined in various ways but at a disciplinary level, it refers to the nature of being (human) and what is considered real and relevant (to a discipline). Without an explicit ontology, that is, without a clear picture of what substantive focuses we value for practice and inquiry, we risk some sense of identity within the discipline and we risk privileging method and other extraneous factors over substance in our inquiry and knowledge development (Yanchar & Hill, 2003).

Metaparadigm

The broadest ontological element is the *metaparadigm*. The metaparadigm is a highly abstract framework that outlines the central focuses of knowledge development in a discipline. The nursing metaparadigm—at least currently—consists of four concepts: person, health, environment, and nursing practice. It is open to change!

The nursing metaparadigm originated in the early 1970s with nurses in education and curriculum development. Lorraine Walker (1971) defined nursing in terms of (1) the persons providing care, (2) persons receiving care for health problems, (3) the environment in which care is given, and (4) the end state of care, well-being. Yura and Torres (1975) then identified four overall themes based upon a survey of 50 BSN programs. They identified the following four concepts: (1) man, (2) health, (3) society, and (4) nursing.

Margaret Hardy, a noted nursing sociologist and philosopher from Boston University, was one of the first nurses to use the term "metaparadigm" in the nursing literature, published in *Advances in Nursing Science* in its inaugural year (1978). She described a metaparadigm as representing the broadest consensus within a discipline about its entities of interest and substantive focus. Then, in an *Image: The Journal of Nursing Scholarship* article, Jacqueline Fawcett (1984) drew from themes published earlier, and from her previous theoretical writings on central concepts of nursing, to formalize the nursing metaparadigm as comprising the four central concepts: person, health, environment, and nursing.

Given these four metaparadigm concepts, we can say that nursing ontology describes beliefs about the nature of human beings and health, the environment, and nursing practice. These concepts are not particularly helpful in guiding knowledge development until they are linked together and elaborated in various conceptual constructions, such as conceptual frameworks and metaparadigmatic statements. For example, Newman, Sime, and Corcoran-Perry (1991) put forth their metaparadigmatic statement: *Nursing is caring in the human health experience.* Historical and contemporary nursing theories and conceptual models are a rich source for learning about nursing ontology and the diversity of perspectives on the four metaparadigm concepts. As part of your philosophical inquiry in the substance of nursing, try developing your own metaparadigmatic statement of nursing.

Worldviews

A second way to understand or clarify your own nursing ontology is to examine the various worldviews used in nursing to frame perspectives about human beings and their health and health care practices. Nursing worldviews may also be called philosophies, discourses, or paradigms. They propose differing beliefs about human beings, health, practice, and other nursing concepts. Some regard worldviews or identification with any overarching perspective as a bias that can corrupt our thinking. Worldviews or "Weltanschauung" typically have been depicted as expressing an implicit, unexamined understanding about the world (Crotty, 1998). But everyone holds some kind of worldview. Articulating our worldviews and critically examining them with openness to other views is a useful process in knowledge development.

Worldviews, in fact, are applied widely across disciplines to understand systems from the cellular to individual to organizational levels. In nursing, worldviews range from mechanistic to developmental views of human health processes, from particularistic to holistic views of person–environment interactions, and from reactive to transformative views of human change. These frameworks originated in various disciplines and fields, including philosophy (e.g., Stephen Pepper's, 1942, *World hypotheses*), lifespan developmental psychology (Lerner, 1986; Reed, 1995), complexity sciences (e.g., see biologist Stuart Kauffman, 1995, and Gaustello, Koopmans, & Pincus, 2009), and nursing (see Fawcett, 1993, for a succinct overview of extant nursing worldviews). Reflecting on your own beliefs and values and/or considering which, if any, worldviews align with your thinking is a form of philosophical inquiry. Doing this can help uncover areas of interest for research as well as expose biases that influence your path to knowledge development.

EPISTEMOLOGY

Epistemology refers to the study of the nature of knowledge, including what is warranted as scientific knowledge in a discipline. Epistemological views have implications for selecting methods of theory development and research on the discipline's subject matter.

Several *patterns of knowing* are involved in producing nursing knowledge, for example, personal, practice, and ethical approaches with patients and families; empirical approaches that include scientific inquiry (Carper, 1978); sociopolitical approaches that inform nurses about sources of oppression in society and science (White, 1995); and emancipatory knowing that reveals injustices and why they endure, and what might be done to remove them (Chinn & Kramer, 2008).

Patterns of knowing may be used together to generate a theory. Alternatively, as Fawcett, Watson, Neuman, Walker, and Fitzpatrick (2001) suggested, each pattern may be used to generate a specific kind of theory, for example, empirical theory or ethical theory. Overall, nurses employ a diversity of research methods to obtain quantitative and qualitative data about the complex domain of nursing phenomena.

Epistemological views are also expressed in *philosophies of science*. These philosophies relate to how problems of study are conceptualized, and underlie methods of research and theory development.

PHILOSOPHY OF SCIENCE

The path to knowledge development is influenced by our philosophies of science. Philosophy of science is a field of study focused on the nature and practice of science, and the growth of scientific knowledge, including the formulation, justification, and evaluation of scientific theories. The field consists of philosophies of science that propose differing beliefs about science and truth, knowledge and reality, and how all of these are related. And as with philosophy of nursing, philosophies of science may constrain our thinking, but they also enable our knowledge development, or "what we call facts to be known, what we call reality to be brought forth and experienced" (Smith, 2005, p. 59). So, clarifying your philosophy of science is a crucial, if not pivotal, event along this path of knowledge development.

There are many philosophical views regarding science described in the literature. Not all are elaborated here, for example, critical theory, critical social realism, and postcolonialism. Major philosophies of science that have influenced science and knowledge development in nursing include positivism, postpositivism, constructionism, and postmodernism. These have emerged across the history of science.

A SHORT HISTORY OF SCIENCE

The path to knowledge changes over time as individuals, societies, and cultures change. And some historians suggest that we cannot say one perspective is better than another at achieving "truth." Understanding something about the history of science as it relates to your philosophy of nursing provides a context for you to clarify your own preferred philosophy of science.

From the 11th to the 15th centuries, scientists (who were mostly astronomers) worked to align their observations with the accepted theory based on the Aristotelian geocentric view of the universe (Oakley, 2000). Interestingly, science began by looking outward far away from earth, and then worked inward toward human affairs (Magee, 2001). The path was mostly anti-empirical and followed the methods of scholasticism; people did not study nature but instead employed logic, reason, and argument to understand and interpret the wisdom in the theology of the sacred texts and the philosophical views of the ancient Greeks such as Plato and Aristotle.

The key to modern science was a shift from testing ideas by argument and discussion to testing ideas by direct observations, measurement, and experimentation (Ferris, 2010; Losse, 2004). The Aristotelian and religious worldviews of the Middle Ages gave way to the new scientific and heliocentric worldviews of the 16th century. The progression of modern science was fueled significantly by 17th century artisans working away with their own hands and ideas (Conner, 2005). Francis Bacon (1561–1626), mathematician and philosopher, is widely attributed with founding the scientific method that would launch modern science, but Conner (2005) reminds us that the evolution from earlier to modern approaches in knowledge development also occurred among the people in their daily practices of their work, generating indigenous knowledge that benefitted society.

A critical mass of thinkers occurred in the 18th century, building on the foundations of knowledge development from 17th century mathematicians and scientists as represented in the following events: the rationalism of Descartes, the scientific method and separation from metaphysics by Bacon, the abstractionism and mechanical discoveries about the universe by Newton, and the empiricism of John Locke. Knowledge was based on what could be "proved logically, tested scientifically, or verified empirically" (Ritchie, 2010, p. 3). This excluded other ways of knowing that derived from art, literature, religion, or personal insight. And it reinforced divisions between rationality and feeling, propositional truth and experience, verifiable history and personal meaning. Science during this time was built on the study of closed, physical systems, which were amenable to mathematical calculations, assumptions about invariant natural laws, and making precise predictions.

Positivism

The scientific revolution of the 17th century helped foster 18th century enlightenment ideas about social progress, human reason, and intellectual freedom. Also during this time, positivism emerged as a philosophy of science in part through the demarcation of scientific discourse from other ways of knowing. It promised progress toward increasingly accurate causal explanations of the world and the unification of all scientific inquiry. This philosophy was based upon an objectivist epistemology, which holds that meaning and reality exist independent of observers' values. Auguste Comte popularized the term "positivism" to distinguish knowledge that would come by speculation or reference to natural law as opposed to knowledge arrived at by direct experience. Comte and the members of the Vienna Circle held an interest in applying strictly empiricist methods of the natural sciences to the social and human sciences. They were interested not only in knowledge but also in precise methods to obtain knowledge. The tenets of positivism include beliefs in the following events and perspectives:

- Objective reality exists independent of culture and observer
- Truth is based on achieving correspondence between theoretical concepts and observables
- Ability of science to attain value-free knowledge of reality
- Clear demarcation between science and all other ways of knowing, especially that concerning religion
- The context of justification, not the context of discovery, of knowledge is the appropriate concern of science
- Observational evidence is valued over theoretical explanations as a basis for scientific inference
- Knowledge comes principally from experience and inductive reasoning
- Scientific results reveal regularities that can be generalized
- Scientific knowledge is built as theories accumulate in a linear manner

Postpositivism

Additional emphases of logic, mathematics, and the use of language transformed positivism into logical positivism during the early 20th century. Postpositivist scientists challenged and tempered the positivist claims of certitude and precise observations without negating its basic objectivist perspective. That is, postpositivism retained the positivist view of reality as "out there" independent of human experience. The tenets of postpositivism state the following:

- Theory and data are not separable; theory influences perception of the "facts"
- Truth is based on achieving theories' correspondence with a reality that is observable yet cannot be fully known
- Science produces inexact knowledge about reality
- Observational evidence underdetermines scientific theories
- Conjecture and deductive reasoning are used in theory development
- Theories are tested by falsification, not verification
- Scientific results are probabilistic
- There are many paths (and methods) but still only one truth, one reality

Twentieth-century discoveries led scientists to question some of their positivist assumptions. For example, discoveries, during the 1920s, in physics about the structure of the atom and scientists' inability to determine the position of subatomic particles with accuracy stimulated questions about their views of reality, the nature of these particles, and science. Scientists began to realize that there was a gap between what they could directly verify by observation and the entities and concepts described in their theories. Their objects of study were too fast, too large, or too small to be directly observed (e.g., electromagnetism, gravity, evolution, embryo, and ego) and description of these proposed entities required conceptual innovations. Scientists began to realize that they were more actively constructing scientific knowledge than they were passively "receiving" it from nature above.

The noted postpositivist philosopher Karl Popper proclaimed that all observation takes place within the context of theory and is shaped by theory. The *received view,* coined by Hilary Putnam to describe the relationship between the reality and the theorist, became the *perceived view*, to emphasize the role of perception in observing reality. The scientist and historian Thomas Kuhn (1962) put forth the idea that scientists in fact make sense of the world by looking through a conceptual apparatus called paradigms, which are based in history and change over time. By the 1960s, these and other influences weakened the dominance of objectivist epistemology, although vestiges still remain in science today, along with constructionist views of reality and knowledge.

Constructionism

Constructionism rejects the view that there is an objective truth and observable reality *out there*, waiting to be discovered. Meaning and knowledge are not discovered but rather are constructed through social interactions between people and between person and environment. Nevertheless, as one writer pointed out, Kuhn's paradigm-shifting revolutions did not completely remove the relevance of science done under a previous paradigm; space shuttles still fly according to Newton's laws (Ferris, 2010).

From *constructionism,* we understand that theory development is a product of social processes between people and their environment (e.g., between the researcher and participants, nurse and patient, the nursing discipline and society). Theory involves interpretation and meaning-making out of our observations. Basic tenets of constructionism include the following:

- Science is a process rather than an event of linear progress
- Knowledge is a product of social interchanges among people, their environment, and culture
- Truth is influenced by nonobservational factors (e.g., social, psychological, historical) that influence the context of discovery, as well as the empirical factors under study
- Acceptable theories achieve coherence within a system of knowledge
- A diversity of research methods are used to study social processes
- Historical and cultural influences are realities of research
- Scientists eschew foundational views but depend upon shared ideas and values
- Knowledge is built by consensus across paradigms
- The practitioner is obligated to confront pragmatic implications and to justify why something is meaningful or useful rather than to justify whether it is true

Postmodernism

Popper and Kuhn's critiques of positivist science "somewhat unwittingly" laid the foundation for postmodernism (Ferris, 2010, p. 247). In postmodernism, science is regarded as a culturally influenced approach that is not necessarily any better than other forms of discourse (e.g., poetry and fiction) in conveying truths (Ferris, 2010, pp. 247–249). Postmodernism resists description. Crotty (1998) applied the epistemological view of subjectivism to describe the relationship between theorist and reality underlying postmodernism as well as poststructuralism, a perspective that is related to, but distinct from, postmodernism. Subjectivism emerged in the latter half of the 20th century. In subjectivism, meaning is imposed on the focus of study by the inquirer. Meaning does not emerge out of the interaction between people but instead emerges more from within (Crotty, 1998). Not all postmodernists adhere to this subjectivist view. Some are especially concerned with the detrimental effects that one's inquiring or scientific gaze has on another.

Postmodernism cannot be summed up in a list of tenets. There are many differences across philosophical views. In general, however, postmodernists eschew four key ideas that are found in either or both postpositivism or constructionism:

- Foundationalism—in *epistemology*, a belief in an unchanging foundation or one view of truth
- Essentialism—in *metaphysics*, the view that people have an "essence"—characteristics that constitute universal features of human nature
- Realism—in *metaphysics*, the belief in a reality that exists independent of historical or social context
- Representationalism—in *philosophy of language,* the view that neither scientist nor artist can reproduce or "mirror" reality. Postmodernists may employ a method called *deconstruction* (from poststructuralism) to reveal the "foolishness" of modern science attempts to represent reality through research findings

Postmodernism's iconoclastic and pluralistic attitudes opened up new possibilities for nursing knowledge development (Reed, 1995). This philosophy of science helped dislodge nurses from dichotomous thinking about science and art, qualitative and quantitative data, empirical and spiritual, facts and values, and theory and practice. This process is not unlike the interpretive method of the hermeneutic circle, where one spirals back and forth between dichotomous or contradictory elements (e.g., part and whole, what is understood and what is not understood, illness and wellness) to gain better understanding of a concept or situation. Nurses entertain the possibility of multiple interpretations, meanings, and methods in knowledge development, and with all scientists of modern philosophical views, postmodernists share a value for skepticism; an enthusiasm for discovery; and a desire for emancipation from ignorance, prejudice, and oppressive authority.

Judd (2009) explains that even Bacon (1561–1626), philosopher and founder of the modern scientific method, was an exemplary model for breaking the rules in the interest of knowledge development. Bacon's empirical method and spirit of experimentation separated him from the beliefs of medieval church scholars and Aristotle's principles of natural philosophy to inspire liberal intellectual thinking in a new practice of science.

INTERMODERNISM: A PLACE BETWEEN *MODERNISMS*

As we travel around the path from Philosophy of Nursing and Philosophy of Science, let's stop just before the next turn where *philosophy* transitions into *action* to consider one final philosophical perspective as it relates to our efforts to produce nursing knowledge. The postmodern discourse on science may have led you to question the value of traditional scientific approaches in knowledge development, if not to construe science itself as a hegemonic practice incongruent with nursing's humanistic and holistic goals. It is not uncommon to read that the terms "postmodernism" and "science" together create an oxymoronic phrase! The two discourses do have some distinct differences. However, the use of reason, questioning, and skepticism that drove the scientific revolution of the 17th century is still valued today, and helps science to endure as a critical, open, and reflective practice that generates knowledge for a discipline. Nevertheless, I suggest that we extend our thinking to consider a place *between* modernisms—between modern and postmodern views—that may better fit 21st century nursing and support practices of nursing science not represented by the other paradigms. I call this perspective *intermodernism.*

Intermodernism builds on an initial formulation of a philosophy of nursing science called *neomodernism* that I presented several years ago (Reed, 1995, 2006), and some have since applied this perspective to advanced practice, science, and research (e.g., Arslanian-Engoren, Hicks, Whall, & Algase, 2005; Liehr & Smith, 2007; Whall & Hicks, 2002).

Intermodernism is a heterodox philosophy of science in that it departs somewhat from traditional views yet finds wisdom in existing philosophies. The term "intermodernism" indicates an approach that does not abandon useful categories of science yet creates a space for us to think about what features we would like or need in a philosophy of science to facilitate knowledge development through our practices of science and nursing care.

Intermodernism is reflected in the overall structure of the spiral path as well as in each element in the path. This is depicted by the arrow in Figure 1.2. The entire knowledge process represented by the spiral path—the nonlinear, nonhierarchical arrangement of elements; the absence of an end point and the openness of theorizing; and the distinct yet merged areas of practice, science, and theory—all emanate from an intermodern view of knowledge development.

You may construct a diagram depicting your own view of the structure of nursing knowledge, identifying the dominant perspective that ties together the various elements, or you may substitute new terms where mine sit on the spiral. The primary intent is to encourage thinking and theorizing among nurses about the question, "*How does that which we call nursing knowledge come into being?*"

The intermodern path accounts for various contingencies that postmodernists informed us about in our search for truth, the unavoidable influences on our theorizing and knowledge development. The turns of the path represent a number of these—for example, personal beliefs; life experiences; socioeconomic factors; and professional experiences, expertise, and worldview—and are regarded as opportunities to enrich rather than constrain knowledge.

THE MIDDLE WAY

Intermodernism is a new term to describe a philosophical perspective of nursing science, but it does not veer too far off the familiar path of science and knowledge

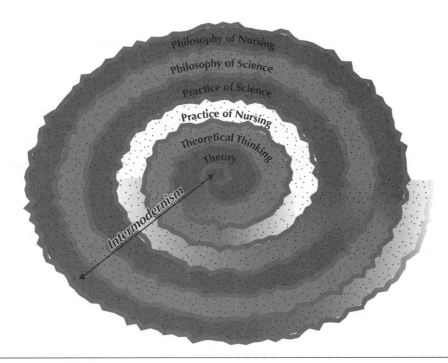

FIGURE 1.2

Intermodernism and the Spiral Path of Nursing Knowledge Development.

development. It honors the wisdom of the middle way. Intermodernism bridges the limitations of a strictly modern view and a strictly postmodern view of knowledge and science. There is an increasing number of scholars from various disciplines attempting to bridge modernism and postmodernism, to broaden approaches to knowledge development beyond boundaries of postpositivism but without the nihilism or other limitations of postmodernism (Mouzelis, 2008). These disciplines include biology, economics, fine arts, literature, psychology, and several health care fields such as health promotion and occupational therapy.

The intermodern view maintains a focus on the person (and other living systems or organizations) as having innate value, emotional and moral senses, and other internal attributes, yet acknowledges the reality of contextual influences (e.g., historical, political, sociocultural) on individuals, families, and communities.

Intermodernism is similar to post-postmodern views, which preserve strands of stability while avoiding radical extremes (Hickman, 2007). Post-postmodernists "tend to be interested in political philosophy, taking democracy and its ideals as a model for addressing philosophical issues." They are pluralist in outlook, but also value "disciplinary structure in scholarship. Fields such as epistemology, theology, philosophy of science, and the history of ideas," which were marginalized by postmodernism, have gained renewed interest (*Routledge Encyclopedia of Philosophy*, 2000, pp. 700–701).

The middle way is pluralistic, encouraging a diversity of ideas. Intermodernism avoids some of the extremes in postmodern philosophy found, for example, in

Kuhn's *revolutions* and Foucault's *ruptures* (Smith, 2005). Through paradoxical rather than dialectical thinking, differences in theories and methods can coexist without being resolved into one synthesis. Instead of the Kuhnian perspective that paradigms are incommensurable and therefore logically must compete through revolution for scientific progress to occur (Stepin, 2005), pluralism allows for new thinking; different paradigms and theories can coexist and still undergo change without being integrated or subsumed into one right view.

However, intermodernists are not so pluralist to the point of relativism where they fail to identify with some shared values in their science community and commit to a common paradigm to facilitate knowledge development, if even within the nurse's particular practice or academic community. Shared values, for example, include personal autonomy, self-development, agency, humanism, and justice.

PATTERN IN THE UNIVERSE

Insofar as at least one universe of nursing is the human system in the context of health-related events and experiences, intermodernism affirms that despite some postmodern proclamations to the contrary, the perception or belief in an underlying order is a foundation of the practice of science. Scientific inquiry is based, in part, upon the idea that there exist laws, tendencies, or patterns inherent in the phenomena of interest to a discipline. Scientific progress is related to the extent that a discipline's theories describe and explain these phenomena and help solve conceptual and practical problems.

Moreover, Carter and New (2004) suggested that the positivist aim to discover universal laws has been exaggerated since many of the laws are not invariant but rather refer to "tendencies" or probabilities that events will occur according to a given principle. Whether you believe that order or pattern resides in nature, in the perceived object, or in the perceiving subject depends upon your philosophical views about the natural and social worlds, and other values and beliefs. These views, in turn, will influence the methods you use in your practice of science to build or test nursing knowledge.

The following are 11 tenets of the intermodern perspective:

- In-between-ness: Theorists work in-between modernism and postmodernism, between extremes and contradictions, yet somehow outside of traditional methods. Thinking can be "[r]adical without being revolutionary, eccentric without being trivial" and is valued for its "departure from 'high' modernism ..." (Bluemel, 2004, p. 66).
- Nursing: Acknowledges modernist descriptions of nursing as a practice and a scientific body of knowledge, but also defines nursing ontologically as inherent processes of well-being within and among human systems (Reed, 1997). Understandings of nursing go beyond modernist descriptions that separate the practice of science from the practice of nursing care to conceptualize nursing as a process that may occur (1) externally in interactions with professional

nurses to facilitate well-being or (2) individually and even internally where person's themselves engage their inner resources for well-being.

- Truth: Defined neither by theories' *correspondence* with one source of truth nor necessarily by theories' *coherence* with a cluster of other theories, but through the *coordination* of multiple theoretical ideas focused on addressing a similar problem. In addition, local truths are valued but an external "corrective" or paradigm is regarded as useful in determining just what is emancipating, good, healthful, and other value-laden truths used in nursing. In this way, nursing offers a "grounded" hope, unlike some postmodernists who offer an "ungrounded hope" from a highly relativist view of truth (Hickman, 2007).

- Empiricism: A new empiricism based on a broadened perspective of what comprises nursing evidence. It includes both objective and subjective data and valorizes the perspectives of patients and families as central in the discovery and justification of knowledge. In addition, there is a network of human, non-human, and hybrid elements that informs knowledge development (Latour & Woolgar, 1986).

- Reality: Found neither "out there" independent of the thinker (realist) nor completely within the thinker's mind (idealist). Rather, reality emerges and acquires its specificity *through* the practitioners' interactions and actions in health care and knowledge development. Acknowledges an underlying pattern, diversity, and innovation.

- Methods: Systematic methods are important to the scientific enterprise, but it is also recognized that science is a messy process, a "mangle of practice" (Pickering, 2005), a fact illuminated by the field of science studies. Knowledge development in nursing practice then exemplifies both the systematic and messy nature of science.

- Openness: Being open to critique, self-correction, and change and an ongoing reflection on one's theory and practice are essential in knowledge development. Openness is congruent with the open, self-organizing nature of human systems in process with their environments.

- Discovery: The context of discovery—the dynamic situations and influences under which knowledge is created—achieves an importance much greater than it had in modern science, which focused on the context of justification of theories. Discovery involves multiple ways of knowing that inform and extend empirical knowing. Abductive reasoning, which is more than the mere combination of inductive and deductive logic, is a dominant pattern of practitioners. Scientific "findings" are constructed more than discovered, but they are "neither arbitrary nor are they constructed out of nothing" (Hickman, 2007, p. 28).

- Epistemology: Promotes a new and expanded epistemology in which science and practice partner to create knowledge. There is a reimagining of practice in the context of theory as a *source* not just as *repository* of knowledge. Practice is a pattern of knowing that informs empirical knowing and knowledge development. Knowledge development is pragmatic and performative, found in experience and in the doing, as well as in the reflecting and thinking. Technology provides new tools; instruments; equipment; machines; biotechnology; and other means for observing the unobservable, for facilitating wholeness in a posthuman culture, and for generating nursing knowledge (and "thing knowledge"; Baird, 2004; Locsin, 2009) about nursing processes that promote well-being.

- Romanticism: Recognizes the reality of the human quest for meaning, goodness, and beauty. Metaphysical views are included in what are considered focuses for empirical study and theorizing in nursing. Spirituality and purpose in life, for example, can be studied empirically as expressions of human experiences related to well-being. Embraces both the scientific view and belief in an ever-present mystery in what can be known (Raymo, 2008; Tauber, 2009). Nonepistemic (social, cultural, emotional) as well as epistemic (having to do with knowledge) values are involved in scientific inquiry. Human beings and indeed the universe are simply too complex and broad to be fully understood by common-sense observation or objectivist scientific study.
- Nightingale: A scientist and scholarly practitioner, and a symbol to remind us to strive for the following events: (1) reclaim the health and unitary focus of person–environment and inner healing capacity espoused by Nightingale; (2) value and build upon nursing's indigenous knowledge, found in classic theorists and scholars, and in lay persons in their everyday health experiences; (3) decolonize our discipline of practices and paradigms that rob nurses of opportunities to build knowledge and provide care from a nursing perspective of health, illness, and end-of-life.

This list of tenets of intermodernism is not necessarily complete. You may think of other potential tenets as you continue to read and reflect. In the following, notice the presence of this philosophical perspective in the final sections on The Practice of Science, The Practice of Nursing, and Theoretical Thinking. There are other examples of intermodernism in knowledge development throughout other chapters as well. Intermodern ideas permeate this book. You may extend this list of tenets as you discern them in your studies and your work in nursing.

THE PRACTICE OF SCIENCE

The practice of science refers to the systematic methods and strategies of knowledge development commonly used in research. The practice of science in the context of nursing care will require generating new scientific methods, for example, from theories of complex adaptive systems, and refining or modifying older qualitative methods such as grounded theory methodology to be more applicable to the complex environment, interactions, and activities that occur in practice. Regardless of the method used, it is understood that no data are "raw" in the modern sense (as direct indicators of reality, pure and devoid of influences) and that science is a mangle of social processes (Pickering, 2005).

Scientific discovery is "an extended process consisting of cycles of generation, evaluation, and revision" (Darden, 2009, p. 53). The close relationships among theory generation, evaluation, and revision show that the positivist distinction between the contexts of discovery and justification is not a useful one. It follows, then, that construction of a distinction between knowledge generation and knowledge evaluation to distinguish between PhD and DNP education and roles, respectively (American Association of Colleges of Nursing, 2004), may be a misguided principle in the practice of nursing science; this potentially could restrain nursing's full capacity for knowledge development.

WEARING TWO HATS: RESEARCHER AND PRACTITIONER

In 20th century nursing, science was modern and clean, or so it seemed. It was clear: Nurses wore only one hat at a time and did not confuse their roles of clinician or researcher—and more often, a nurse always only wore one hat, with the nurse researcher developing the knowledge that was then handed down to the clinician to apply in practice. However, as Latour (1993) explained, *we have never been modern*. New thinking about knowledge development in nursing brings scientific inquiry and nursing practice together more closely where nurses' observations and interactions with people in health-related situations provide opportunities for knowledge development, testing, and evaluation. But the complexity of nursing care requires creative and new approaches to knowledge development.

One reason for this complexity is that the phenomena of central concern to nursing—human beings and their health-related processes and experiences—is not easily divided for education and practice purposes into basic and applied focuses between the bench scientist and clinical practitioner. Contexts of nursing practice, that is, places where nurses interact with patients to promote health or where people engage their own health processes to help themselves heal, are also laboratories of nursing science. Because we do not easily divide the human being and health experiences into parts, our discipline cannot easily make coequal divisions, for example, between the scientists and engineers, or bench scientists and practitioners—and the practices of knowledge development cannot be separated into basic, foundational science versus the applied, technological knowledge.

ENGINEERS, NURSES, AND INNOVATION

In elaborating on the innovative thinking of engineers in his latest book, Petroski (2010) elaborates a description of the engineer that can be applied to the practitioner scholar in nursing: It is the engineer's ability not just for the "observational and predictive thinking" used in traditional science, but for "conceptual and constructive thinking" that creates new knowledge in the context of engineering problems (p. 15). Granted, all knowledge builds upon foundational conceptual knowledge and past theories in some way, but the innovative and original knowledge of engineers that Petroski (2010) champions reaches beyond the translation or application of knowledge produced by the bench science of the physicist or chemist. The knowledge developed by the engineer "cannot be taken off nature's shelf; they are *pure creations* of engineering" (author's emphasis, Petroski, 2010, p. 22).

So, there is a nonlinear relationship between the practice of science and the practice of nursing care that fosters the emergence of new knowledge. As with Galileo's discoveries with the telescope, practice advanced science. Galileo's practice with the telescope provided the needed context to (1) improve the telescope and (2) lead the way to scientific understanding of (and theorizing about) underlying principles. The pragmatics and problems of practice stimulate the practice of science. As Petroski (2010) explained, "Pure science and pure truth are things of the past." Science is no longer "unfettered by practical concerns" free to pursue natural phenomena not connected to practice (p. 114). He witnessed that the linear model of R&D (*Research and Development*) has been reversed (*Development and Research*). And so it may be with the practice of science in the discipline of nursing, given a new emphasis on what Petroski (2101) labeled "real-world directed research" (p. 118). Solutions to problems involving complex systems will require involvement of complex systems of knowledge development. The theories generated by practicing nurses must go beyond that based on traditional principles and laws. "Principles may inspire...but they do not create the situation or structure" needed to develop knowledge (p. 174).

Thus, the practice of nursing science involves use of systematic methods to examine, evaluate, refine, and extend theoretical ideas. Theories will identify important concepts but also reach beyond description of concepts or assessment of clinical phenomena to elucidate new connections. The practice of science in the 21st century will likely involve designing new ways to gather and analyze clinical data to inform our theorizing.

THE PRACTICE OF NURSING

In looking at the spiral path, you will notice that there is no clear demarcation between the practice of science and the practice of nursing. This is the reality of practice-based knowledge development. The practice of nursing is an art of combining the contingencies of the moment, including diverse patterns of knowing, with systematic and scientific knowledge to create a caregiving situation. Similarly, Georgia O-Keeffe created her works of art from an inner creative vision but also knew the science of her practice, that is, the technical skills, methods, and basic theoretical concepts of composition, balance, and color.

And out of a nurse's caregiving situation theory can emerge. This is the central thesis of this chapter and book. That is, with ample reflection on practice situations coupled with their fund of clinical knowledge and some understanding of theories and theory development, nurses can produce compelling knowledge in practice! This may be more easily done than explained. "Theory is created at the moment of action through a complex, and as yet inadequately understood, process of reflecting in action" (Clarke, James, & Kelly, 1996, p. 176). An intermodern conceptualization of the practice-theory link differs from modernist views of nurses who were expected to act on theories formed prior to the practice without reference to the particular practitioner or context. However, scholars were not any clearer in explaining how knowledge was produced in practice 15 years ago when nurses were expected simply to apply theory to practice.

Knowledge development in practice is like Neurath's boat image: Otto Neurath was a philosopher of science who likened theory building to the rebuilding of a ship at sea:

> *We are like sailors who have to rebuild their ship on the open sea, without ever being able to dismantle it in drydock and reconstruct it from the best components. (Neurath, 1983, p. 92).*

His image does little to elucidate the process of knowledge development in practice except to emphasize the inextricable link between theory and practice.

INQUIRY INTO KNOWLEDGE DEVELOPMENT IN NURSING PRACTICE

A few scholars have taken on the challenge of explaining practice-based science and practice-based theory development, creatively extending Dickoff and James's (1968) classic thesis on "practice theory" (e.g., Diers, 2004/1985; Doane, Browne, Reimer, MacLeod, & MacLellan, 2009; Doane & Varcoe, 2005; Kim, 1993, 1999). These efforts are on the rise. From an intermodern stance, the question behind this challenge is not the classic epistemological concern *"What is nursing knowledge?"* but instead *"How does that which we call nursing knowledge come into being?"* The answer requires philosophical, ethical, and empirical inquiry.

The answer will not be found by the modern approach to theory that dichotomizes knowledge production and application research in educating doctoral nurses, practitioners, academicians, or administrators. The answer is not found in using the discourse of *application* when relating theory and practice. The applied idea for moving theory into practice worked when we held a postpositivist of science, which separated or at least attempted to separate knowledge development and knowledge use, science and values, the context of discovery and the context of justification, mind and body, health and health care, science and technology, theory and practice, and nursing and practice.

The answer will be found beyond (modern) notions of theory, with new interactions between nurses' practices of science and nursing care. Much more research into contexts of health caregiving as contexts of discovery will be needed to address empirical, epistemological, and ethical issues that arise when practicing nurses practice science. Practice is an undertheorized context of knowledge development (Rolfe & Gardner, 2006).

TRANSFORMING PRACTICE KNOWLEDGE INTO NURSING KNOWLEDGE

Although practice is an undertheorized context of knowledge development, Peplau's (1952, 1988) classic works provide excellent insights into how knowledge and theory may be generated in practice. Peplau was known for her theory on the interpersonal relations published in 1952. However, what many nurses do not know of Peplau is her *cycle of inquiry* whereby she described practice as a process of transforming practice knowledge into nursing knowledge.

Peplau presented the nurse–patient relationship as a context for conceptual innovations. Her strategy for practice-based inquiry has some similarity to that described by contemporary scholars (Brown, 2009). A key point is building on existing knowledge and theories while bringing in new ideas from clinical experiences to *innovate* concepts for theory development. Existing theories provide a base for developing and evaluating new ideas. Knowledge builds on itself.

Peplau's Cycle of Inquiry[1]

Nursing practice typically has been viewed as a context for *applying* but not *developing* knowledge, but the therapeutic relationships that are integral to nursing practice are also a means for testing and building theory. Peplau's work elevated nursing practice to the level of scholarship; that is, she connected nurse–patient interactions to theoretical ideas and concepts. She synthesized ideas from theories of Sullivan, Maslow, and Fromm. Yet her approach to inquiry for nursing let the patient and the "voice of nursing" (Johnson, 1993) be heard above the theory. In doing this, Peplau introduced an approach to knowledge development that was anchored in nursing practice, and in the science and art of the nurse–patient interaction. Development and testing of explanations through the interpersonal process between patient and nurse were done for therapeutic purposes—but, according to Peplau, this interpersonal process was also a strategy for generating nursing knowledge. Steps 1, 2, and 3 describe her strategy of transforming practice knowledge into nursing knowledge. These steps, incidentally, are also an early example—ahead of its time—of abductive thinking in developing nursing knowledge.

STEP 1: OBSERVATION OF FUNDAMENTAL UNITS. Knowledge development, according to Peplau, begins with observations made in the context of practice. For Peplau, this context was primarily the nurse–patient relationship. Observation preceded conceptual interpretations. Peplau (1952) outlined various methods of observation that yielded knowledge, including spectator observation, role-playing, and random observation. However, Peplau (1952, 1992a) emphasized participant-observation, in which a nurse uses self as both the instrument and object of observation while participating in the interpersonal process with a patient.

According to Peplau, a nurse enters a situation with theoretical understanding, personal bias, and previously acquired nursing knowledge. Patients enter with their knowledge and with the powers and capabilities of a developing human being. Patients possess the principle data for inquiry in the form of underdeveloped or unused competencies, subconscious meanings, and personal knowledge. Nurses possess knowledge of methods to help patients make use of their competencies and to regain well-being.

---

[1] Portions of this text were adapted from Reed (1996) with permission from John Wiley & Sons.

Peplau (1992b) explained that, while on a "philosophical level" human beings may not be reducible, elements about human beings can be studied and measured to develop nursing knowledge at the "theoretical level" (p. 88). Scientists and scholars agree that knowledge production, at least in part, involves placing boundaries around phenomena. Relevant "units of observation" according to Peplau are those that are meaningful and useful to patients, measurable, and definable, and that can be replicated and compared with other data (Peplau, 1952, p. 270). Fundamental units of inquiry within Peplau's theory (1952, 1988) are *processes* and *patterns* and the *problems* that can emerge from them.

Processes refer to behaviors that develop over time in observable phases (Peplau, 1987, 1992a). She included nursing therapeutic processes, such as the four-phased interpersonal relationship, as that which "co-operates with and assists" other processes to move the patient toward health (p. 125).

Patterns are comprised of separate thoughts, feelings, or actions that share the same theme or aim (Peplau, 1987, 1992a). Patterns that are shared by two or more people are called "pattern-integrations," and they may be mutual (when both parties exhibit the same set of behaviors), complementary, or antagonistic.

Thus, building knowledge entails observation of human processes and patterns, fundamental units of study. The *problems* that arise from these may also be studied, while drawing from knowledge about the underlying processes and patterns to produce theoretical explanations.

STEP 2: PEELING OUT AND TESTING THEORETICAL EXPLANATIONS: PEPLAU'S ABDUCTIVE APPROACH. Once initial observations are made by a nurse in an interpersonal relationship, theoretical concepts are then "peeled out" and drawn into the interpersonal process to explain observed phenomena (Peplau, 1973; Letter to Geraldine Ellis cited in Welt & O'Toole, 1989; Peplau, 1988). This process is not unlike abductive reasoning described in the section on Theoretical Thinking. *Peeling out* refers to abstracting concepts from clinical knowledge and from existing scientific theories and conceptual frameworks; these concepts represent the phenomena observed in practice, and are subsequently connected together in a logical way to formulate a conceptual or theoretical framework. Peplau (1988) identified this as part of a nursing process of "interpreting observations." This process includes such investigative activities as creative invention, decoding, subdividing data, categorizing data, identifying layers of meaning at different levels of abstraction, and applying a conceptual framework to explain phenomena.

Through "peeling out," hypotheses are drawn from the nurse's observations (Peplau, 1952, p. 269). These tentative explanations that are formulated are then validated with the patient and tested for their meaningfulness and usefulness in the context of the nurse–patient relationship.

Peplau's theorizing was not limited by a strict adherence to formulating operational definitions or deducing testable statements from existing "high theories." Rather, Peplau's regard for universal patterns in psychosocial development, learning, and other human experiences was tempered by her emphasis on the clinically based reality created during encounters with patients (Reed, 1996).

STEP 3: TRANSFORMING ENERGY AND TRANSFORMING KNOWLEDGE. The final step is application of theoretical knowledge through interactions with patients. This results in the transformation of practice knowledge into nursing knowledge. The term "application" hardly captures this transformation, because it requires aesthetic perspective, intellectual competencies, and clinical judgment (Peplau, 1988, p. 13).

The test of the truthfulness of knowledge, according to Peplau (1952; 1988), was not based upon how well the knowledge corresponded to a preexisting theory but how effective it was in helping patients enhance their self-understanding and developmental progress. Nursing knowledge is developed in the context of practice through synthesis of (1) existing scientific theories, clinical observation, and judgment of nurses, and (2) knowledge and active participation of the patients. Thus, Peplau's interpersonal process provides a context for engaging in both nursing care (helping the patient to transform anxiety into productive energy) and nursing science (peeling out theories, testing them, and in so doing, transforming practice into nursing knowledge.)

NURSING KNOWLEDGE

In Peplau's (1952) cycle of inquiry, nursing knowledge that is generated through nursing practice is further evaluated and refined through research methods. The resulting knowledge becomes part of a practicing nurse's repertoire of nursing knowledge, which undergoes transformation and validation in subsequent nurse–patient encounters, as the cycle of inquiry begins again.

During the early modem era of nursing, nursing researchers often borrowed knowledge from other disciplines to be passed on to the practitioners. However, Peplau's (1952) cycle of inquiry produced practiced-based nursing knowledge rather than borrowed knowledge. It is *nursing* knowledge by virtue of its link to nursing processes and nursing practice. In sum, Peplau's cycle of inquiry provides a classic perspective on nursing practice as more than a context for applying a tested and refined theory: Practice is a context for initiating and testing theory.

THEORETICAL THINKING

Theoretical thinking, identified near the center of the figure, really spirals through the entire journey of the path. It is an ever-present practice. All disciplines have theories and engage in theoretical thinking. In fact, everyone has working theories about how they view their world and how things function. Children create their own theories to explain how and why things occur. Adolescents and adults do this as well. Practitioners think theoretically to make sense of their everyday encounters. It is the scientists who are unusual in regard to theorizing—they have explicit rules about how to develop theories, how to use them, and how to judge their theories.

Theoretical thinking is the basis of our humanity. It is in our ability to "make theories, to test them from experience, and then make new and better ones, that intelligence emerges" (Gopnik, 2009, p. 186). Gopnik explained that the scientists' ability to theorize reflects a person's ability to continue to learn, to be open to new thinking, and to define the world in new ways. This ability, he says, brings dignity to those who make theories.

All thinking is impregnated with theory, especially our scientific conceptualizations. Ferris (2010) explained that we are now so enlightened about the presence of theory that we tend to mock the 17th century idea that science is merely the sum of observations and take for granted our realization that facts and observations are theory laden. Gopnik (2009), in his publication about Darwin's work, explained that "it is in the jump beyond, to a general rule, a theory, even a vision, that science advances."

ABDUCTIVE REASONING

Theoretical thinking in nursing, and particularly nursing practice, may be described largely by the process of *abduction*. Abduction was first described by philosopher of science Charles Peirce (1934) and then elaborated by Hanson (1958) to propose a form of reasoning involved in discovering a plausible explanation, inferring a hypothesis, or generating a theory. This form of reasoning is the third but most important form of logic, next to inductive and deductive logic. Abduction generates more substantial knowledge than can either deduction or induction alone.

With abduction, the theorist brings together observation and theory, experiences and existing knowledge, to posit a potential explanation for a given situation or event. The nurse takes a creative, conceptual leap to posit possible reasons or underlying processes to explain its occurrence—and the explanation may extend beyond what is readily observed at the present time; the abduction creates a holding place for evidence that may be found later, with improved empirical methods or technology, for example, to better explain the underlying process (Weissman, 2008). Nurses characteristically mistake their abductive reasoning for the mysteries of intuition! Nurses in practice often must act upon their best judgment in the absence of perfect knowledge—making simultaneous connections between their keen observations and interactions with patients and extant theories and other patterns of knowing—to produce knowledge for action. Recognizing this expertise for theoretical thinking may enable nurses to more deliberately produce theoretical knowledge out of their practice encounters.

Abductive reasoning produces open theories. The practitioner uses new data and ideas as they arise to test and modify or refine the theory. There are several sources in the literature that outline examples, details, and steps in abductive thinking (e.g., Montgomery, 2006; Råholm, 2010; Weissman, 2008), although most focus on knowledge development by the researcher rather than the practitioner. Nevertheless, it is likely to be the new generation of doctoral nurses with *all* kinds of doctoral nursing degrees who will describe abductive thinking for knowledge development by practicing nurses!

CHAMPIONING THEORETICAL THINKING TO SUSTAIN A DISCIPLINE AND ILLUMINATE PROCESSES

For nurses in particular, theoretical thinking provides the disciplinary focus and basis of our practice. And theorizing helps nurses understand the clinical phenomena with which they deal everyday. By theorizing, nurses create a mental image of a concept or an event—to see, to ponder, to understand, and to communicate with others, and then use in practice in some therapeutic or meaningful way (Thorne, 2005). By theorizing, practitioners make sense of their daily lives.

Disciplines share knowledge and borrow theories from other disciplines. However, the strength of a profession's jurisdiction in practice and the clarity of a discipline's identity and contribution to society are dependent upon the explication of a discipline's own theories (Abbott, 1988; Potvin & Balbo, 2007). A key characteristic of both a science and a profession is having theories that are unique to that discipline. More specifically, the mark of scholarship in nursing practice is not the practice alone but when "the intellectual work [of the nurse]…raises the clinical instance to the level of theory" (Diers, 2004, p. 84). Both the conceptual and the empirical are valued.

Theories have important functions in a practice. Kurt Lewin (1951) is often quoted, "there is nothing as practical as a good theory" (p. 169). Theoretical thinking moves knowledge forward by imagining new concepts and mechanisms occurring in practice. "It is in the leap of the data, not the heap of the data…[where] the advance lies" (Gopnik, 2009, p. 71). Knowledge developed in the form of theory does not merely describe a situation or concepts in isolation; it links concepts, ideas, and events to each other to propose some underlying process.

The contemporary writer, bell hooks' (1999) description of writing relates to theorizing in practice: We do it "to find secrets in experience that are obscured from ordinary sight: to uncover hidden coherences in what seems to be a mere jumble of unrelated events and details, and to find incoherence in what appears to be strictly ordered; to make transparent what is opaque, and to expose opacity in what seems transparent" (p. 40). So, theories give us new perspectives, sensitize us to what patients are saying, and help us to listen in new ways and discover new ideas that can be of greater help to patients. And when our theories cannot fully explain, they can offer up abstract concepts, as a place holder for things we cannot quite grasp while we forge ahead in knowledge development, rebuilding our ship as we sail the seas.

Theoretical thinking reflects the middle way of intermodernism in that it involves analysis and interpretation, systematic thought and imagination. Theorizing is not the result of simply employing analytical thinking and a logical, standardized procedure. Nor is it a process of unplanned flashes of insight (Meheus & Nickles, 2009). It takes a little of both, plus adequate doses of creativity, imagination, and perseverance. Theories help us avoid errors from two extremes, of narrow empiricism that limits our sights to one way of knowing and "unanchored abstract thought" that attempts to explain all (McQueen, 2007, p. 22).

THEORY

Theory resides in the center of the spiral path. This position is not an end point but a place that launches the nurse back through the path to test out and refine theoretical knowledge. Theories consist of concepts and proposed relationships between concepts. They provide explanations of processes proposed to underlie or influence phenomena of interest to a discipline.

Nursing theories are emergent products of a nurse's personal experiences and beliefs, professional activities and practices, philosophy of nursing, and philosophy of science, as well as the skill and strategies nurses use in developing knowledge. Theories are open to critique and change. Writers who disparage theory (e.g., Thomas, 2007) offer worthwhile critique but often criticize from a positivist, and therefore limited, view of theory. Theories provide perspective, specificity to inform action, distinction, and clarity for one's professional identity and also provide a (relatively) secure base from which to connect and collaborate with other disciplines in practice and research.

Theories are practical in that they provide an efficient structure to frame our questions and from which to interpret the findings. Good theories help identify the factors to be studied and the questions to be asked. Theories are like clinical or research instruments; they make evidence "observable" that would otherwise be inaccessible (Weissman, 2008), while at the same time being open to testing and change as more clarity is achieved.

DESCRIBING THEORY

Theories are organizations of nursing concepts and evidence into conceptual structures that help practitioners and researchers see pattern and organization in their activities and make sense of what they observe and discover in their work. Theories by definition have both empirical and abstract dimensions. They consist of concepts and statements of relationships between concepts that point to not only a local process or event but also a possible pattern of which the local event is one example. A theory is a tool for conceptualizing and studying practice problems, proposing explanations and interventions, and testing and refining ideas.

Types of Theories

Theories come in different sizes, so to speak. These range from *conceptual models* and *grand theories* that are broad in scope and focus on a large domain of nursing, to *middle range theories* that address a focused area of research or practice in a discipline, to *microlevel theories* that have the narrowest scope and most specific focus (see Higgins & Moore, 2000, for a succinct overview).

Middle range theories are the most common theories in science. They have less scope than grand theories or conceptual models, and instead focus on specific health experiences, health and illness problems, or certain patient populations.

They are still relatively abstract yet provide some explanations about nursing phenomena. Middle range theories have concepts that can be defined empirically so that the relationships proposed in the theory can be tested or explored empirically, through systematic approaches in practice or other settings. Theories are tested by deriving research questions or hypotheses (propositions) from the theory for testing. Nurses build knowledge by testing theories against observations of the natural world, in practice and elsewhere. *Testing,* from an intermodern perspective, reflects evaluative values (discussed later) that are somewhat different from values promoted in modernist science.

Theory as a System

Theories also can also be thought of as a system, with a boundary and system conditions, interrelated parts internal to the system, and elements that are external to the system that influence its development (Dubin, 1978). The spiral path has outlined several of these external elements that influence theory, such as the nurse's philosophy and practice. *Modern* perspectives depict the relationship between practice and theory as linear, one of dissemination of theory to practice. *Intermodernism* depicts a different relationship. It is nonlinear, one of transformation where both are changed by the relationship between theory and practice. The relationship is one of transformation rather than dissemination (Latour, 1993). It is important to note that theory and practice are distinct processes because in that way they can generate the change that fosters knowledge development. As a system, then, a theory is dynamic and open to change through research, debate, critique, and through its expression in practice.

Theory as Process and Product

THEORY AS A GIFT. As a process, theory is a scholarly way of thinking that stimulates new ideas and illuminates potential connections between ideas. But more than this, theory is a process of interacting with patients in practice, which generates the ideas that are formulated into theories. Theory, then, may be regarded as a gift, given by the situation or encounter with patients in nursing care. The nurse's theorizing, in turn, is a way of appreciating the gifts given by patients, a form of appreciative inquiry.

Nature writer and scholar, Kathleen Dean Moore (2010), explained that in living close to the wilderness, she had to learn to accept its gifts—and the way to learn, she said, was to practice. She did this by giving back, through her writing about nature. Nurses too, live close to wilderness and nature in their daily practice with patients and families. The insights, ideas, and lessons that nurses acquire through their work are gifts. They arise from any place where nursing is practiced—in health-related interactions with patients and their families, colleagues, students, teachers, friends and family, and in quiet self-reflection. Nurses give back not only through their practice but also by developing the potentialities of the caregiving interactions into theories of new knowledge.

THEORY AS AN ART FORM. As a product, theory can be viewed as an art form. Eisner (1985) said that "all scientific inquiry culminates in the creation of form: taxonomies, theories, frameworks, and concept systems. The scientist, like the artist, must transform the content of his or her imagination into some public, stable form, something that can be shared with others …" (p. 26). In this way, theory is viewed as a product that proposes and shares possible explanations or solutions. Nursing theories have a particular form and substantive focus, often providing insights and interpretations on one or more of nursing's metaparadigm concepts. The art of theory involves an abstraction from the concrete experience to inform us about a *pattern* (not just a *part*) of human health.

Theories as Nets

A modern or postpositivist view of theories portrays them as nets tossed out to the sea to catch a part of reality. We cannot catch the entire ocean, so an important first step in theory development is to clarify what part of the ocean is our focus (our ontology), and our methods (epistemology) for designing and deploying our net. The nature of the netting will influence the kind of "truths" that are caught from the ocean. Moreover, an intermodern view of theories regards the nets *as* reality. "The net, a web of shifting, intersecting, interacting beliefs and practices, *is* truth" (Ludwik Fleck cited in Smith, 2005, p. 51). Our theories, then, are quite powerful in influencing our experiences and practices with patients.

EVALUATING THEORIES

Evaluating theories is an important process in the path of knowledge development. As dynamic, humanly constructed structures, theories need to be evaluated by a complex set of criteria. Evaluation criteria are useful in judging the merits of a theory and may also be used to guide the development of a theory. These criteria typically reflect both epistemic values (which are concerned with justifying the theory as true and accurate) and cognitive, social, or moral values (which also warrant the knowledge but in a manner connected more closely to the social dimension of science.) Standard values from modernist science include empirical adequacy, parsimony, coherence, generality, predictability, broad scope, fruitfulness, and objectivity. From an intermodern perspective of knowledge, which is pluralistic in its approach to differing values, the list of criteria includes selected standard criteria (e.g., empirical adequacy) as well as new criteria, all of which are believed to support the aims of science. The following list, then, proposes new considerations of several standard criteria for evaluating theories (Longino, 2008):

- Parsimony may be modified to allow for *complexity* to better capture the complex and dynamic nature of a human system or situation.
- Coherence may be modified to value *novelty* in a theory so that theories do not necessarily have to be consistent with existing theories and the status quo. Theories that offer new understandings are desired over accepted theories that perpetuate older views not appropriate or useful in the present context.

- Generality and scope of a theory may be purposely *limited* or focused so as to explain patterns unique to a given situation, case, health experience, or group of people, for example.
- Fruitfulness or pragmatic adequacy, which typically focuses on a theory's ability to generate new *research* problems, may be modified in practice situations to focus on a theory's capacity to alleviate human needs and promote health empowerment.

Overall, then, we do not necessarily want criteria that promote homogeneity and unity in nursing knowledge and theories. There is rarely one causal factor or even one stable set of factors that explains health processes and experiences. Human beings, who comprise nursing's major focus, are complex and dynamic. Where traditional science calls for criteria that help screen out alternative theories to arrive at the one best theory, we often need a pluralism of theories to explain nursing phenomena. This can happen only if practicing nurses, as well as other participants in scientific inquiry, join together in the production and evaluation of nursing theories.

TOWARD A NETWORK OF SCHOLARS

Van den Daele (2004) explained that since the 19th century, modern science progressed as the "implicit and embodied knowledge of the practitioner [was replaced] by the explicit and disembodied knowledge of the scientists" (p. 34). However, he goes on to warn that the traditional scientists' vision for knowledge development may be too narrow for the increasingly complex nature of society. "In dealing with complexity, the limits of the *knowing scientists* may be narrower than the limits of the *knowing practitioner*, for instance in handling human life and behavior, organizations, or technical systems" (p. 34). Clearly, the wisdom of the practitioner along with other nurses will be needed to build the knowledge and theories of the 21st century.

According to 20th century modernist practices of science, nursing research and practice were regarded as separate domains: Scientific knowledge was developed by the researchers and then handed down through mechanisms variously called dissemination, application, or research utilization to practicing nurses. Postmodernist ideas spread in the later third of the 20th century and challenged traditional thinking across many disciplines about knowledge generation. The movement stimulated new ideas about the relationship between theory and practice and who should participate in defining truth for a discipline. Shifts in thinking about knowledge development and practice are still unfolding in this century.

As a discipline rich with practice, theory, and research dimensions, nurses can be *thought leaders* in knowledge innovations that advance societal welfare. Nursing science and practice employ multiple patterns of knowing and views of truth while still valuing certain foundational principles first expressed in the grand theories. Nurses are embracing multiple methods of theory development and research, and a pluralism of theories that inform nursing interactions. Classic theories are still appreciated for their historical significance in distinguishing nursing among other health care disciplines and as a foundation for knowledge development, but new ideas about theory and knowledge development are on the horizon—ideas generated by the knowledge potential inherent in the burgeoning of doctoral nurses who will enter practice as well as academe and other scholarly positions in the next decade. Nursing theories will have to be accessible, flexible, and responsive to the knowledge needs of practicing nurses and the public. Theory will not so much be applied or disseminated from research to practice as it will emerge from scholarly thinking in practice, and then continue to be transformed as practice contexts change.

Theories are windows for the world to peer in to the knowledge of disciplines. *What knowledge will enter the world through nursing?* Nursing has an increasing number of doctoral level practicing nurses who will become an untapped resource for knowledge development if they are not educated into the knowledge building process. Historians of science tell us emphatically that to sustain our profession, knowledge must become disciplinary; that is, there must be an ongoing and organized core of like-minded individuals who work together in building knowledge into useful and meaningful theories of that discipline. Our large and complex discipline needs a network of strategies and a network of scholars for knowledge.

Knowledge development draws from philosophical, empirical, and theoretical dimensions of nursing knowledge. A scholar sees all practices as inquiry, always asking why, yet appreciating the mystery, and always reaching for new ideas—whether predominantly as a practitioner, philosopher, scientist, theorist, teacher, or learner. We need nursing scholars in all practices who can walk the path of inquiry to build nursing knowledge. Engaging and educating practicing nurses more deliberately, along with other graduate nurses, in theory development will provide nursing with a more sustainable approach to fostering knowledge for our future health care needs.

QUESTIONS FOR REFLECTION

1. How has this chapter helped you to answer the question, "How does that which we call nursing knowledge come into being?" From your experiences, do you have ideas about this that were not presented in this chapter?
2. How do you see the Path as influencing your participation in building nursing knowledge?
3. What component(s) of the Path were most helpful in understanding how nursing knowledge can be developed? Which components of the Path left you with questions?
4. Eleven tenets of intermodernism were proposed. How closely do you identify with the perspectives of this new philosophical view? Do you disagree with some tenets?
5. How has this chapter helped you begin to think about your own theory innovations through your nursing practice or research?

REFERENCES

Abbott, A. (1988). *The system of professions*. Chicago, IL: University of Chicago Press.

American Association of Colleges of Nursing. (2004). *Position Statement on the Practice Doctorate in Nursing*. Washington, DC: AACN.

Arslanian-Engoren, C., Hicks, F. D., Whall, A. L., & Algase, D. L. (2005). An ontological view of advanced practice nursing. *Research and Theory for Nursing Practice: An International Journal, 19*(4), 315–322.

Baird, D. (2004). *Thing knowledge: A philosophy of scientific instruments*. Berkeley, CA: University of California Press.

Bluemel, K. (2004). *George Orwell and the radical eccentrics: Intermodernism in literary London*. New York: Palgrave Macmillan.

Brown, H. I. (2009). Conceptual comparison and conceptual innovation. In J. Meheus, & T. Nickels (Eds.), *Models of discovery and creativity* (pp. 29–41). New York: Springer.

Carper, B. (1978). Fundamental patterns of knowing in nursing. *Advances in Nursing Science, 1*(1), 13–23.

Carter, B., & New, C. (Eds.). (2004). *Making realism work*. New York: Routledge.

Clarke, B., James, C., & Kelly, J. (1996). Reflective practice: Reviewing the issues and refocusing the debate. *International Journal of Nursing Studies, 33*(2), 171–180.

Chinn, P. L., & Kramer, M. K. (2008). *Integrated theory and knowledge development in nursing* (7th ed.). St. Louis, MO: Mosby.

Concise Routledge Encyclopedia of Philosophy (2000). New York: Routledge.

Conner, C. D. (2005). *A people's history of science: Miners, midwives, and low mechanics*. New York: Nation Books.

Crotty, M. (1998). *The foundations of social research*. Thousand Oaks, CA: Sage.

Darden, L. (2009). Discovering mechanisms in molecular biology: Finding and fixing incompleteness and incorrectness. In J. Meheus & T. Nickles (Eds.), *Models of discovery and creativity* (pp. 43–55). New York: Springer.

Dickoff, J., & James, P. (1968). A theory of theories: A position paper. *Nursing Research, 17*(3), 197–203.

Diers, D. (2004). Clinical scholarship. In D. Diers (Ed.), *Speaking of nursing...narratives of practice, research, policy and the profession* (pp. 79–89). Boston: Jones and Bartlett Pub. (Reprint from Diers, D. (1995). Clinical scholarship. *Journal of Professional Nursing, 11*(1), 24–30.)

Doane, G. H., Browne, A. J., Reimer, J., MacLeod, M., & MacLellan, E. (2009). Enacting nursing obligations: Public health nurses' theorizing in practice. *Research and Theory for Nursing Practice: An International Journal, 23*(2), 88–106.

Doane, G. H., & Varcoe, C. (2005). Toward compassionate actions: Pragmatism and the inseparability of theory/practice. *Advances in Nursing Science, 28*(1), 81–90.

Dubin, R. (1978). *Theory building* (Rev. ed.). New York: The Free Press.

Eisner, E. (1985). *Learning and teaching the ways of knowing*. Chicago, IL: University of Chicago Press.

Fawcett, J. (1984). The metaparadigm of nursing: Present status and future refinements. *Image: The Journal of Nursing Scholarship, 16*(3), 84–87.

Fawcett, J. (1993). From a plethora of paradigms to parsimony in worldviews. *Nursing Science Quarterly, 6*, 56–58.

Fawcett, J., Watson, J., Neuman, B., Walker, P. H., & Fitzpatrick, J. J. (2001). On nursing theories and evidence. *Journal of Nursing Scholarship, 33*(2), 115–119.

Ferris, T. (2010). *The science of liberty: Democracy, reason, and the laws of nature.* New York: HarperCollins.

Fromm, E. (1947). *Man for himself.* New York: Rinehart.

Gaustello, S. J., Koopmans, J., & Pincus, D. (2009). *Chaos and complexity in psychology: The theory of nonlinear dynamical systems.* New York: Cambridge University Press.

Gopnik, A. (2009). *Angels and ages: A short book about Darwin, Lincoln, and modern life.* New York: Alfred A. Knopf.

Hanson, N. R. (1958). *Patterns of discovery: An inquiry into the conceptual foundations of science.* Cambridge: Cambridge University Press.

Hardy, M. E. (1978). Perspectives on nursing theory. *Advances in Nursing Science, 1*(1), 27–48.

Hickman, L. A. (2007). *Pragmatism as post-postmodernism: Lessons from John Dewey.* New York: Fordham University Press.

Higgins, P. A., & Moore, S. M. (2000). Levels of theoretical thinking in nursing. *Nursing Outlook, 48*(4), 179–183.

Hooks, B. (1999). *Remembered rapture: Writer at work.* New York: Henry Holt & Co.

Johnson, R. (1993). Nurse practitioner-patient discourse: Uncovering the voice of nursing in primary care practice. *Scholarly Inquiry for Nursing Practice, 7,* 143–158.

Judd, D. M. (2009). *Questioning authority: Political resistance and the ethic of natural science.* New Brunswick, NJ: Transaction Pub.

Kauffman, S. (1995). *At home in the universe: The search of laws of self-organization and complexity.* New York: Oxford University Press.

Kim, H. S. (1993). Practice theories in nursing and a science of nursing practice. *Scholarly Inquiry for Nursing Practice: An International Journal, 8*(2), 145–162.

Kim, H. S. (1999). Critical reflective inquiry for knowledge development in nursing practice. *Journal of Advanced Nursing, 29*(5), 1205–1212.

Kuhn, T. (1962). *The structure of scientific revolutions.* Chicago, IL: University of Chicago.

Latour, B. (1993). *We have never been modern* (C. Porter, Trans.). New York: Harvester Wheatsheaf.

Latour, B., & Woolgar, S. (1986). *Laboratory life: The construction of scientific facts* (2nd ed.). Princeton, NJ: Princeton University Press.

Lerner, R. M. (1986). *Concepts and theories of human development* (2nd ed.). New York: Random House.

Lewin, K. (1951). *Field theory in social science: Selected theoretical papers.* New York: Harper & Row

Liehr, P., & Smith, M. J. (2007). A neomodernist perspective for researching chronicity. *Archives in Psychiatric Nursing, 21*(6), 345–346.

Locsin, R. C. (2009). 'Painting a clear picture': Technological knowing as a contemporary process of nursing. In R. C. Locsin & M. J. Purnell (Eds.), *A contemporary nursing process: The (un)bearable weight of knowing in nursing* (pp. 377–394). New York: Springer Pub.

Longino, H. E. (2008). Values, heuristics, and the politics of knowledge. In M. Carrier, D. Howard, & J. Kourany (Eds.), *The challenge of the social and the pressure of practice: Science and value revisited* (pp. 68–86). Pittsburgh, PA: University of Pittsburgh Press.

Losse, J. (2004). *Theories of scientific progress.* New York: Routledge.

Magee, B. (2001). *The story of philosophy* (2nd ed.). New York: Dorling Kindersley Pub.

Maslow, A. (1954). *Motivation and personality.* New York: Harper & Row.

McQueen, D. V. (2007). Critical issues in theory for health promotion. In D. V. McQueen & I. Kickbusch. (2007). *Health and modernity: The role of theory in heath promotion* (pp. 21–42). New York: Springer.

Meheus, J., & Nickles, T. (Eds.). (2009). *Models of discovery and creativity.* New York: Springer.

Montgomery, K. (2006). *How doctors think: Clinical judgment and the practice of medicine.* New York: Oxford University Press.

Moore, K. D. (2010). *Wild comfort: The solace of nature.* Boston: Trumpeter.

Mouzelis, N. P. (2008). *Modern and postmodern social theorizing: Bridging the divide.* New York: Cambridge University Press.

Neurath, O. (1983). Protocol statements. In O. Neurath (Ed.), *Philosophical papers: 1913–1946* (pp. 91–99) (R. S. Cohen & M. Neurath, Ed. and Trans.). Boston: D. Reidel Pub Co.

Newman, M. A., Sime, A. M., & Corcoran-Perry, S. A. (1991). The focus of the discipline of nursing. *Advances in Nursing Science, 14*(1), 1–6.

Oakley, A. (2000). *Experiments in knowing: Gender and method in the social sciences.* New York: The New Press.

Peirce, C. S. (1931–1958). *Charles Sanders Peirce: Collected papers* (Vol. 1–6), C. Hartshorne & P. Weiss (Eds.) (Vol. 7–8), A. W. Burks (Ed.). Cambridge, MA: Harvard University Press.

Peplau, H. E. (1952). *Interpersonal relations in nursing.* New York: Putnam.

Peplau, H. E. (1987). Interpersonal constructs for nursing practice. *Nursing Education Today, 7*(95), 201–208.

Peplau, H. E. (1988). The art and science of nursing: Similarities, differences, and relations. *Nursing Science Quarterly, 1*, 8–15.

Peplau, H. E. (1992a). Interpersonal relations: A theoretical framework for application in nursing practice. *Nursing Science Quarterly, 5*, 13–18.

Peplau, H. E. (1992b). Perspectives on nursing knowledge (interview by T. Takahashi). *Nursing Science Quarterly, 5*, 86–91.

Pepper, S. P. (1942). *World hypotheses: A study in evidence.* Berkeley, CA: University of California Press.

Petroski, H. (2010). *The essential engineer: Why science alone will not solve our global problems.* New York: Alfred A. Knopf.

Pickering, A. (2005). *The mangle of practice: Time, agency and science.* Chicago, IL: University of Chicago Press.

Potvin, L., & Balbo, L. (2007). From a theory book to a theory group. In D. V. McQueen & I. Kickbusch (Eds.), *Health and modernity: The role of theory in heath promotion* (pp. 6–11). New York: Springer.

Råholm, M. (2010). Abductive reasoning and formation of scientific knowledge within nursing research. *Nursing Philosophy, 11*, 260–270.

Raymo, C. (2008). *When God is gone everything is holy: The making of a religious naturalist.* Notre Dame, IN: Sorin Books.

Reed, P. G. (1995). A treatise on nursing knowledge development for the 21st century: Beyond postmodernism. *Advances in Nursing Science, 17*(3), 70–84.

Reed, P. G. (1996). Transforming practice knowledge into nursing knowledge—A revisionist analysis of Peplau. *Image: Journal of Nursing Scholarship, 28*(1), 29–33.

Reed, P. G. (1997). Nursing: The ontology of the discipline. *Nursing Science Quarterly, 10*(2), 76–79.

Reed, P. G. (2006). Neomodernism and evidence based nursing: Implications for the production of nursing knowledge. *Nursing Outlook, 54*(1), 36–38.

Reed, P. G. (2010). The spiral of nursing theory. *The Japanese Journal of Nursing Research, 4*(2), 87–92.

Ritchie, D. E. (2010). *The fullness of knowing: Modernity and postmodernity from Defoe to Gadamer.* Waco, TX: Baylor University Press.

Rogers, M. E. (1970). *An introduction to the theoretical basis of nursing.* Philadelphia: Davis.

Rolfe, G., & Gardner, L. (2006). 'Do not ask who I am …': Confession, emancipation and self-management through reflection. *Journal of Nursing Management, 14,* 593–600.

Sibeon, R. (2007). An excursus in post-postmodern social science. In J. L. Powell & T. Owen (Eds.), *Reconstructing postmodernism: Critical debates* (pp. 29–40). New York: Nova Science Pub.

Smith, B. H. (2005). *Scandalous knowledge: Science, truth and the human.* Edinburgh, England: Edinburgh University Press.

Stepin, V. (2005). *Theoretical knowledge* (A. G. Georgiev & E. D. Rumiantseva, Trans.). Dordrecht, The Netherlands: Springer.

Sullivan, H. S. (1947). *Conceptions of modern psychiatry.* Washington D.C.: William Alanson White Psychiatric Foundation.

Suppe, F. (1977). *The structure of scientific theories* (2nd ed.). Chicago, IL: University of Illinois Press.

Tauber, A. I. (2009). *Science and the quest for meaning.* Waco, TX: Baylor University Press.

Thomas, G. (2007). *Education and theory: Strangers in paradigms.* Berkshire, England: Open University Press.

Thorne, S. (2005). Conceptualizing in nursing: What's the point? *Journal of Advanced Nursing, 5*(2), 107.

Van den Daele, W. (2004). Traditional knowledge in modern society. In N. Stehr (Ed.), *The governance of knowledge* (pp. 27–40). New Brunswick, NJ: Transaction Pub.

Walker, L. O. (1971). Toward a clearer understanding of the concept of nursing theory. *Nursing Research, 20,* 428–435.

Weissman, D. (2008). *Styles of thought: Interpretation, inquiry, and imagination.* New York: SUNY Press.

Welt, S. R., & O'Toole, A. W. (1989). Hildegard E. Peplau: Observations in brief. *Archives of Psychiatric Nursing, 3,* 254–264.

Whall, A. L., & Hicks, F. D. (2002). The unrecognized paradigm shift in nursing: Implications, problems, and possibilities. *Nursing Outlook, 50,* 72–76.

White, J. (1995). Patterns of knowing: Review, critique, and update. *Advances in Nursing Science, 17*(4), 73–86.

Yanchar, S., & Hill, J. R. (2003). What is psychology about? *Journal of Humanistic Psychology, 43*(1), 11–31.

Yura, H., & Torres, G. (1975). Today's conceptual framework within baccalaureate nursing programs. In National League for Nursing (Ed.). *Faculty-curriculum development, Part III: Conceptual Framework—Its meaning and function* (pp. 17–25). New York: National League for Nursing.

Doctoral Nursing Roles in Knowledge Generation

Donna M. Velasquez
Donna Behler McArthur
Catherine Johnson

*I*t has been nearly a decade since the Institute of Medicine (IOM, 2003) called for "a major overhaul" in the way heath care professionals are educated to meet the challenge of improving health care in the 21st century. This challenge has resulted in sweeping changes in health care education including the creation of two new educational degrees for nursing, the Clinical Nurse Leader and the Doctor of Nursing Practice (DNP). The American Association of Colleges of Nursing (AACN) has described the goal for DNP education as a "transformational change in education required for professional nurses who will practice at the most advanced level of nursing" (AACN, 2006, p. 4).

As of June 2010, there were 127 DNP programs enrolling students in the United States, with an additional 100 programs planned (AACN, 2010). A number of factors have contributed to the burgeoning number of programs offered in the United States, including the endorsement of moving the current level of preparation for advanced nursing practice from a master's degree to the doctorate by 2015. However, despite the increased number of programs and over 600 graduates (AACN, 2010), there remains a great deal of confusion about the role of the DNP graduate within nursing and other health professionals.

Graduates of DNP programs are described as expert practitioners who possess a wide array of knowledge and have the ability to apply and translate evidence into practice (AACN, 2006). However, as noted by Smith and McCarthy (2010), the vision for practice, described in the *Essentials of doctoral education for advanced nursing practice* (*DNP Essentials*; AACN, 2006), is not much different than how advanced nursing practice has "been envisioned for the past several decades, except for the emphasis on the new knowledge outside of the discipline ..." (p. 49). While application of knowledge is at the philosophical core of practice doctorates such as the DNP, there is little discussion of the role of the DNP graduate in the generation of new knowledge from practice. Simply applying knowledge generated by others is not a "transformational change in education" but rather a continuation of the old paradigm. Individuals with the capability of generating and applying knowledge provide organizations with a sustainable competitive advantage (Nonaka, Toyama, & Konno, 2000). A needed change in education is to foster generation of knowledge from practice as well as translation and application of knowledge. This change is mandated, given our struggle to meet demands for high quality care in a rapidly changing health care environment with decreasing financial resources.

DNP education is at a crossroad between the creation of an essentially entry-level degree (such as the MD, JD, and PharmD) or creating a truly transformational and terminal doctoral degree. In this chapter, we explore the role of the DNP graduate in relation to the role of the PhD-prepared nurse. We also propose a conceptual model on the distinct and shared contributions to the generation and application of knowledge by the DNP-prepared nurse as practitioner–theorist–researcher (PTR) and the PhD-prepared nurse as scientist–theorist–researcher (STR).

EVIDENCE-BASED PRACTICE AND BEYOND

The nursing practice doctorate program leading to the DNP degree is designed to prepare experts in specialized advanced nursing practice. The DNP title does not designate a specialty, rather DNP graduates will be prepared for a variety of roles including leadership, administration, and advanced practice nursing (nurse practitioners, clinical nurse specialists, nurse anesthetists, and nurse midwives; AACN, 2006, p. 8). DNP programs have two entry levels: post-baccalaureate and post-masters. The focus is on practice that is innovative and evidence based, reflecting the application of credible research (AACN, 2006, p. 3). The goal of evidence-based practice (EBP) is to promote effective nursing interventions, efficient care, and improved outcomes for patients, and to provide the best available evidence for clinical, administrative, and educational decision making (Newhouse, Dearholt, Poe, Pugh, & White, 2007, p. xiv).

EBP: HISTORY AND MODELS

Early models of research utilization predated the EBP movement and should be appreciated as exemplars in narrowing the research–practice gap. Perhaps the best known project was the CURN Project (Conduct and Utilization of Research in Nursing) conducted by the Michigan Nurses' Association in the 1970s (Horsley, Crane, & Bingle, 1978). The goal was to increase the use of research findings in the practice of registered nurses within 20 hospitals. Findings supported that utilization of research was relevant to practice. The Stetler/Marram Model of Research Utilization (Stetler, 1994) was designed for the application of knowledge (instrumental, conceptual, and symbolic) and can be applied at the individual or institutional level.

Sackett, Rosenberg, Gray, and Richardson (1996) describe evidence-based medicine (EBM) as ancient in its origins, yet a relatively young discipline "whose positive impacts are just beginning to be validated" (p. 312). The term "EBM" has been adopted by many disciplines including nursing and is more commonly referred to as evidence-based practice. Early criticism (and one that continues) included the equating of EBP with "cook-book" medicine. However, EBP goes beyond the mere adherence to published guidelines to combine thoughtful and systematic appraisal of multiple sources and levels of evidence with the integration of the individual provider's clinical expertise and the patient's values and preferences (Melnyk & Fineout-Overholt, 2005).

Models of EBP have continued to emerge since the early 1980s including the Rosswurm-Larrabee Model of EBP (Rosswurm & Larrabee, 1999), the Iowa Model of Research in Practice (Titler et al., 2001), the ACE Star Model of EBP (Stevens, 2004), and the Johns Hopkins Nursing EBP Model using the Practice Question, Evidence, Translation process (Newhouse et al., 2007). While purposes of the models vary, they all help the nurse organize thinking about how knowledge advances from basic discovery to application in practice whether at an organizational or individual level. Shared components of all models are determination of an identified need; data gathering; decision to accept, modify, or reject evidence; implementation; and evaluation. Desired outcomes are to maintain or improve patient health by reducing unnecessary variation in practice and improving quality and safety of care.

Quality of care and patient safety are central to the IOM report *Crossing the quality chasm* (IOM, 2001) and are clearly articulated in the *DNP Essentials* (AACN, 2006) recommendations. Quality improvement (QI) initiatives spearheaded by DNP graduates exemplify building knowledge about local care and methods for improving practice to increase quality and safety within their health care systems. Knowledge production is measured according to its contribution to improved outcomes rather than contribution to generalizable knowledge (Rolfe & Davies, 2009). QI science, unlike basic science designs that often control for contextual factors, works within the local context to study what outcomes are achieved in what settings with what roles and processes. This requires knowledge of the discipline, local culture, QI methodologies, and how to manage change. Unfortunately, most doctorally prepared nurses are more familiar with basic research than with QI science methods (Cronenwett, 2010; Cronenwett et al., 2009) or other methods more suitable to complex and rapidly changing practice environments.

The term *knowledge-to-action* is used to encompass the use of knowledge by stakeholders including practitioners, policymakers, patients, and the public. While many terms are used interchangeably (knowledge translation, knowledge transfer, research utilization, implementation, diffusion, and dissemination) to describe the knowledge-to-action processes, knowledge translation (KT) is the term most generally used in the literature (Graham et al., 2006). KT encompasses all forms of knowing (scientific and other) aimed at increasing the use of knowledge to solve human problems (Estabrooks, Thompson, Lovely, & Hofmeyer, 2006; Graham et al., 2006). A variety of KT models exist including organizational innovation models; social science models of research utilization; research utilization models in nursing; and health promotion models. However, considerable work is still needed to develop and refine theory-based models of KT (Graham & Tetroe, 2007).

GOING BEYOND EXISTING MODELS

Going beyond EBP assumes that nursing students appreciate the concepts of EBP and research utilization taught at the undergraduate and graduate levels. Certainly most health care professionals would agree that care should be delivered based on information about what works. However, the challenge that remains is clarifying what evidence is and how this evidence is used in everyday decision making within the context of clinical practice. Furthermore, how theory and knowledge are generated from practice has not been well articulated.

One characteristic of a discipline is its distinct body of knowledge. This knowledge, however, derives from a variety of sources and ways of knowing. Further, knowledge is not developed in a linear manner. Theory leads to practice, but also practice leads to theory (Boyer, 1990). The outcomes of EBP and KT within unique practice settings and contexts provide potential sources of new knowledge. Relying solely on models of EBP and KT to guide nursing practice, with their emphasis on application of knowledge and their lack of processes for theory building and innovation, limits generation of knowledge. While research-based evidence is necessary for providing optimal care, it is not sufficient (Straus, Graham, & Mazmanian, 2006). Indeed, "... clinical scholarship is more than evidence based practice which can be applied rigidly without passion or creativity. Under certain circumstances, evidence based practice can even be a barrier to innovation" (Pepper, 2010, p. 54).

DOCTORAL DEGREE NURSING AND KNOWLEDGE DEVELOPMENT

Historically, nursing followed the lead of the sciences, medicine, and other health care disciplines in placing highest value on the scientific empirical approach to creating new knowledge. In the 20th century, the philosophy of science that typically undergirded PhD programs emphasized research methods that produced context-free and replicable data. Because of this, many nurses conducted their research farther from the site of practice and from the providers of nursing care. Increasingly however scholars have questioned the relevance of these context-free data (Holloway & Wheeler, 2002; Rolfe, 1998) noting that expert practice involves making decisions within a particular context requiring knowledge from external and "contextual and idiosyncratic evidence" (Avis & Freshwater, 2006, p. 223). The practice doctorate in nursing has helped stimulate movement away from strict adherence to traditional methods of research with new models of clinical knowledge generation and practice being envisioned.

HISTORICAL PERSPECTIVES ON THE PRACTICE DOCTORATE

The MD and biomedical PhD are often used as exemplars of practice and research doctoral degrees. Although there are areas of overlapping knowledge, the MD and PhD students are educated in "radically different ways" and, once graduated, have distinctly different roles (Shulman, Golde, Bueschel, & Garabedian, 2006, p. 29).

As a discipline, nursing has more in common with education as that discipline also struggles to clearly define roles and expectations for research and practice doctorates (PhD and EdD, respectively). The goal of the two doctoral degrees in education is to create equally valuable but distinct degrees with overlapping areas of knowledge. Despite the goal, the EdD does not always garner the same respect as the PhD, and has been referred to as a "low-end PhD" or "PhD-lite." These terms have already been applied to the DNP or as heard at a recent conference "a masters with whipped cream." There is a perception that practice doctorates are an easy option to earning the title of "doctor" (Kirkman, Thompson, Watson, & Stewart, 2007). The confusion of purpose to prepare both researchers and practitioners in education has resulted in neither being done very well (Shulman et al., 2006), and nursing may be in danger of following suit.

The concept of a practice doctorate is not new to nursing. Doctor of Nursing Science (DNS, DNSc) and Nursing Doctorate (ND) programs were introduced in the 1970s as clinical or practice-based degrees. However, with the exception of the ND program at Case Western Reserve University in Cleveland, which is called a DNP program, there is now little difference between most of these early practice doctorates and current research intensive PhD programs (Marion et al., 2003; Patzek, 2010). In an attempt to avoid a repeat of practice-based doctorates transitioning to research degrees, there is an overemphasis on differentiating the two degrees while negating areas of overlap. This is especially apparent where there is an absence of content on philosophy, metatheory, and theory development and evaluation within DNP programs as influenced by the AACN *Essentials of doctoral education for advanced nursing practice* (AACN, 2006). This decreased emphasis places nursing at risk for losing a foundational understanding of the practice of nursing and becoming increasingly influenced by other disciplines (Whall, 2005). Furthermore, the *Essentials* document calls for DNP graduates who are prepared to "Develop and evaluate new practice approaches based on nursing theories ..." (AACN, 2006, p. 9), which, if absent from DNP education, relies on nursing theory taught to students in their undergraduate or master's programs.

A CONCEPTUAL MODEL OF DOCTORAL NURSING KNOWLEDGE GENERATION

To make way for practice-based knowledge generation, a new model for conceptualizing the relationship between nursing research and nursing practice is needed. New models for discipline-based research and practice have emerged in other health care disciplines and are designed to address the educational needs of expert practitioners as well as recognition of the changing research needs important to the discipline (Ragland, 2006; Stephan, 2006).

While tacit knowledge has long been accepted as legitimately created through practice, the significance of practice experiences in developing explicit new scientific knowledge has not been adequately recognized or promoted. This may be due, in part, to the fact that the discipline is still in the process of identifying what and how knowledge-development approaches are used in practice. Nevertheless, we think that practice-based methods of nursing knowledge development require systematic observation, appropriate methodologies, and synthesis of evidence not unlike that required to develop knowledge in academic research settings. However, while basic processes of science are valued and shared by DNP and PhD nurses, there may be important differences in the types of questions and use of methods suitable to complex practice environments. To help advance the idea that practitioners can and should do research, we have proposed a model that clarifies some of the distinctions and similarities between DNP- and PhD-prepared nurses, with particular focus on their roles in development of nursing knowledge. The next step for the near future is to clarify research methods that may be used in practice to build knowledge.

ROLES IN PRACTICE AND RESEARCH

Jarvis (2000) was one of the first to claim that the "practitioner–researcher" model was critical for nursing given the increased emphasis upon efficiencies of nursing practice and the wide spread belief that a gap exists between nursing theory and nursing practice. Freshwater (2003) distinguished between the "practitioner–researcher" and the "scientist–researcher." The scientist–researcher focuses on the development of explanatory, predictive theories to arrive at general statements about large areas of reality. The goal of the practitioner–researcher is problem solving and producing more specific statements about local and contingent situations (Freshwater, 2003, p. 4). We extended these authors' ideas about doctoral nursing roles in our conceptual model to envision how all doctoral nurses may contribute to theory-based knowledge.

In our model, the domain of the DNP-prepared nurse is identified by the term PTR while the domain of the PhD-prepared nurse is identified in the model as STR (see Figure 2.1). The addition of "theorist" in each domain was done to acknowledge that all doctorally prepared nurses, whether predominantly practitioners or academicians, make contributions to nursing theory. This idea of the practitioner as theorist is not new. As Rosemary Ellis explained, if nurses were to move beyond "the personal accumulation of wisdom from patient to patient" (Ellis, 1969, p. 1438), practitioners must be willing to become scholars to develop and test theories derived from practice. Building on this, Reed (2008) advanced the notion of the "practitioner as theorist" introducing new perspectives for developing theory from practice. It is through practice that the relevance of nursing theories is determined. Nurses are educated into understanding that they can apply or adapt existing theories, as well as develop new theories from systematic observations in practice settings to be applied, tested, and ultimately transformed into nursing knowledge (Reed, 2008).

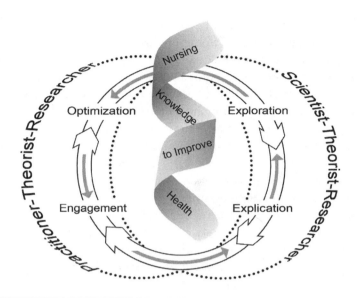

FIGURE 2.1

Conceptual Model of Doctoral Nursing Roles in Knowledge Generation.

The two outer circles in the model (depicted by dotted lines) represent the two domains, STR and PTR, which comprise core roles for knowledge generation. A key dynamic represented by the intersecting circles is the permeability of boundaries between the STR and PTR to not only reduce role constraints but also facilitate knowledge flow between academic and practitioner communities with the creation of partnerships and collaborations. While Baumbusch et al. (2008) and many others have emphasized the reciprocity and exchange between producers and users of knowledge, we propose that being solely a producer or solely a user of knowledge is untenable for doctoral nurses; the STR and PTR alike must participate in knowledge production. PTRs are uniquely positioned to observe firsthand patient responses to health care processes and interventions and therefore, are in a key position to not only apply but also generate new knowledge and theories. Rather than perpetuate the role of the handmaiden, whether to the theory-based knowledge of the physician or to the knowledge produced by the PhD-prepared nurse, the model depicts the PTR as an equal partner in knowledge and theory development to improve human health. Thus, the addition of the PTR role for DNP graduates broadens nursing's resources for knowledge development through distinct, as well as shared, contributions of both doctoral nurse roles.

SYNTHESIZING EXISTING MODELS OF PRACTICE KNOWLEDGE DEVELOPMENT

We developed our conceptual model by synthesizing ideas from the literature as well as through reflection on our own practices. We drew some ideas from two existing models of knowledge development in practice: The ACE Star Model (Stevens, 2004) and translational research models (Woolf, 2006).

The ACE Star Model of Knowledge Transformation (Stevens, 2004) depicts knowledge as evidence from research combined with extant knowledge from other sources and integrated into practice. The stages of knowledge development include knowledge discovery, evidence summary, translation, integration, and evaluation. The emphasis is on transforming large amounts of basic knowledge into a form useful for everyday clinical decision making to improve patient outcomes (Stevens, 2004; Stevens & Staley, 2006).

Several translational research models have been published. For many, the meaning of translational research is limited to the translation of basic science into drugs, devices, and new medical treatments (from bench to bedside) (Woolf, 2006). However, just as EBP is applied widely across disciplines and professions, translational science has application beyond the medical context. Translational research is more broadly defined as the "overarching principle of judicious application of synthesized knowledge to improve health outcomes for individuals and the health care system" (Graham & Tetroe, 2007; Straus et al., 2006; Vincent, Johnson, Velasquez, & Rigney, 2010).

While models of translational research vary in number of steps or stages, all begin with basic or discovery research referred to as T1. T1 research is the focus and recipient of the majority of federal funding and is performed by clinical scientists with mastery of basic sciences (Woolf, 2006). T2 (and additional phases beyond T1 depending on the particular translational model) are concerned with the implementation, evaluation, and dissemination of knowledge to influence everyday decision making by the practitioner. "T2 struggles more with human behavior and organizational inertia, infrastructure and resource constraints, and the messiness of proving effectiveness" (Woolf, p. 212) within complex environments that cannot be neatly controlled.

A strength of EBP and translational models in explicating knowledge-development approaches among DNP- and PhD-prepared nurses is that these models describe processes of advancing knowledge from research to practice. However, the focus in these models is on the application of knowledge handed over from the basic sciences while failing to capture the dynamic process of knowledge and theory generated from practice (Nonaka et al., 2000).

PHASES OF KNOWLEDGE DEVELOPMENT IN PRACTICE

In our conceptual model, knowledge development is proposed to occur across four phases, as identified in the conceptual model: *exploration, explication, engagement,* and *optimization.* Theory and knowledge development are recognized as occurring across all phases—not only in the exploration and explication phases but also continuing into practice as characterized by the phases of engagement and optimization.

Exploration represents the phase of knowledge development that has traditionally been referred to as the process of knowledge discovery (Boyer, 1990).

Theory is generated to explain some phenomenon using conventional research methods to systematically obtain quantitative and qualitative data. Typically, in the Western science paradigm, PhD scholars in academic settings have been recognized as the primary knowledge producers. However, this paradigm is shifting and knowledge production is increasingly viewed as distributed throughout society (Bartunek, Trullen, Bonet, & Sauquet, 2003). Within our conceptual model, this phase represents a primary, but not exclusive, domain of the PhD prepared nurse.

Explication includes testing a proposed theory or interventions under ideal circumstances and where internal validity is a key concern. Explication is somewhat analogous to theory evaluation in which strengths and weaknesses are uncovered through a process of testing and examining outcomes in reality although the "reality" is still closely controlled and effects of context are minimized to increase internal validity. The methods of knowledge development associated with this phase typically have been emphasized more in PhD than DNP curricula. Nursing research has occasionally remained at this phase with few academic researchers having the opportunity to fully integrate knowledge and theory into sustainable practice in context-laden environments.

Engagement refers to the meshing and integration of knowledge into practice. For this phase we employed an extension of the notion of integration presented in the ACE Star Model. Our term of engagement goes beyond the integration of knowledge initially developed through basic research. Engagement describes a dynamic process that implies the commitment of participants to implementation, evaluation, and dissemination of knowledge as it is applied in practice and to the generation of new knowledge from practice. This process requires understanding nursing theory, systems, and methods suitable for complex practice environments. Knowledge and theory are not only applied but are also generated in this phase through action and interaction among individuals and organizations (Nonaka et al., 2000). KT, program evaluation, and QI methodologies are integral to this phase. DNP curricula that emphasize these areas uniquely prepare DNP graduates to use these methods to lead knowledge development.

Optimization is the phase in which knowledge and theory generation is viewed as dynamic and ongoing, continuously inspiring new questions and innovations. Optimization is defined as "an act, process, or methodology of making something (as a design, system, or decision) as fully perfect, functional, or effective as possible" (Merriam-Webster online, 2010). In this phase, external validity is a main concern. Interventions are revised and refined until they are optimal for a specific context, culture, and population. This is an ongoing process requiring a "flexible, responsive, and subjective approach" to knowledge production (Rolfe & Davies, 2009, p. 1271). Through the process of revision and refinement, new questions or problems may stimulate exploration. However, not all problems will require a return to the exploration phase; instead, the knowledge generated in this phase may lead to changes in health policy, or other changes at organizational, unit, or individual levels—all of which capitalize on DNP graduate role preparation.

SUMMARIZING THE STRUCTURAL ELEMENTS OF THE CONCEPTUAL MODEL

Within our model, a central circle depicts the dynamic process of nursing knowledge development that involves research methods used in each of the four phases: *exploration, explication, engagement,* and *optimization.* The process is not necessarily linear as indicated by forward and backward arrows. The forward arrows suggest the traditional notion of knowledge as it is generated and transformed from basic discovery through application and evaluation. However, if there are poor or unexpected outcomes at any phase, there may be a return to the previous phase indicated by backward arrows. The area marked by the intersection of the two circles represents the knowledge generated through the interaction of various methodologies, collaboration and partnerships, and disciplinary knowledge foundational to both roles of doctorally prepared nurses.

Although, the circle depicts an orderly movement of knowledge from one phase to the next, a central spiral is used to characterize the synergy and "messiness" (nonlinearity) that occurs among the stages and across roles. While exploration and explication are primarily viewed as domains of the STR and engagement and optimization the domains of the PTR, boundaries are permeable and flexible as indicated by the dotted lines of the two outer circles. Both nursing roles may engage in any of the methods that constitute the phases. While this flexibility and permeability of roles add complexity in our depiction of knowledge generation, it is really meant to indicate the differences between PhD and DNP educational programs while recognizing that lifelong learning is not bounded to formal degree programs. That is, the PhD- and DNP-prepared nurses may extend their research practices beyond those traditional methods learned in their programs, to learn to use the methods of the *other* knowledge-development domain.

IMPLICATIONS FOR CURRICULUM: PRACTICE-BASED KNOWLEDGE DEVELOPMENT

This proposed model has curricular implications for particular areas of knowledge and skills needed by the "practitioner–theorist–researcher" beyond those typically taught across DNP programs today. The *Essentials for the practice doctorate* (AACN, 2006) emphasizes the scholarly role of the DNP graduate through integration and application of knowledge. However, we maintain that for health care to be transformed, knowledge generated through practice must be legitimized and valorized. The doctoral nursing curriculum is one important place to initiate this movement. Missing from the *DNP Essentials,* the foundation for most programs is the intensive and extensive emphasis on disciplinary knowledge through the study of theory and practice models (Smith & McCarthy, 2010).

Knowledge about the philosophy and theories of nursing science help create a common language necessary for communication within the discipline. Nursing has learned well the language of medicine and other disciplines to enable interdisciplinary collaboration, but there remains a communication gap *within* nursing contributing to the theory–practice gap. An understanding of theory and research as related to knowledge-development practices depicted in the DNP and PhD domains may better enable nursing graduates to translate nursing science as well as other disciplines' scientific knowledge into practice. Furthermore, there is a need to develop theory building strategies that "have fit and relevance in practice" (Reed, 2008, p. 317), which are enhanced by the combined perspectives of the STR and PTR nurses.

Our conceptual model of knowledge and theory generation provides a model for developing curricula to teach the content and skills needed to develop new knowledge through research and practice while continuing to recognize knowledge and theory from other disciplines. Content in the areas of nursing theory, clinical practice expertise, nursing research and evaluation methods, critical reflection skills, expert decision making, and collaboration and networking skills will prepare DNP graduates to more fully assume their role as "practitioner–theorist–researcher." Preparation in these areas will strengthen and broaden nurses' own practice expertise and their ability to contribute theories that inform the discipline and its practices overall.

ENVISIONING THE FUTURE OF KNOWLEDGE DEVELOPMENT AND NURSING PRACTICE

The nature of clinical practice is changing rapidly while the interactions between practitioner and client maintain their uniqueness. Nevertheless, it is within this practice environment that practitioners may creatively synthesize all evidence available to them to construct an approach to the care of their individual patients and unique patient populations. It is also within this environment that relevant pragmatic clinical research is both needed and possible. Every practice engagement between a practitioner and patient has the potential to be an opportunity for research. In addition, purposeful utilization and evaluation of evidence obtained in the clinical setting by the PTR can legitimize the evidence and expand the knowledge base beyond context-free databases.

The goal of the practice doctorate in nursing is to create the highest level of practitioner (AACN, 2006). However, this may entail more attention to developing the tools of scholarship and knowledge development than was originally conceived. "A doctorally prepared [nursing] graduate is expected to both utilize and develop knowledge" (Dracup, Cronenwett, Meleis, & Benner, 2005, p. 179), whether the nurse is prepared with a DNP, PhD, or other nursing doctoral degree. Clinical scholarship practice by the DNP will not be achieved by merely supplementing current master's level curriculums with a few additional courses. Instead, we need entire curricula that incorporate theory, research, and practice methodologies suited to complex practice environments and, at the same time, support development of excellent clinicians. With the growing numbers of students entering BSN to DNP programs there may be increasing numbers who have little background in nursing theory on which to base practice. This is essential in moving EBP from a "cook-book" approach to a conscientious, caring, and scientific process to improve health care.

Our conceptual model proposes a collaborative approach to research in delineating practitioner–researcher and the scientist–researcher roles. Interrelating the two worlds of practitioner–researcher and scientist–researcher expands the possibilities for improving care and, ultimately, improving human health. Both roles are needed to best serve nursing's goal of improved practice. Academic DNP and PhD programs have an opportunity to build models of shared research projects that would not only demonstrate a breadth of knowledge generation strategies but also encourage and guide collaboration among nursing experts. Our conceptual model represents one way to move forward in thinking about the roles of all doctorally prepared nurses in knowledge development for the discipline of nursing.

QUESTIONS FOR REFLECTION

1. In looking at the conceptual model and thinking about your practice experiences,
    • What are some of the challenges that you might face engaging in the roles to build knowledge?
    • What are problems or areas of interest that you would like to see studied in your practice setting?
2. The chapter outlined four phases in knowledge generation, which can be shared by DNP and PhD nurses. What type of questions and methods are suitable for the complex practice environment based on your experience or readings?
3. A collaborative approach to research in delineating practitioner–researcher and the scientist–researcher roles has been proposed in this chapter. How might you use the model in your own practice to move nursing knowledge forward in a new way?

REFERENCES

American Association of Colleges of Nursing. (2006). *The essentials of doctoral education for advanced nursing practice*. Washington, DC: Author.

American Association of Colleges of Nursing. (2010). Amid calls for more highly educated nurses, new AACN data show impressive growth in doctoral nursing programs. Retrieved from http://www.aacn.nche.edu/Media/NewsReleases/2010/enrollchanges.html

Avis, M., & Freshwater, D. (2006). Evidence for practice, epistemology, and critical reflection. *Nursing Philosophy, 7*, 216–224.

Bartunek, J., Trullen, J., Bonet, E., & Sauquet, A. (2003). Sharing and expanding academic and practitioner knowledge in health care. *Journal of Health Services Research & Policy, 8*(S2), 62–68.

Baumbusch, J. L., Kirkham, S. R., Khan, K. B., McDonald, H., Semeniuk, P., Tan, E., et al. (2008). Pursuing common agendas: A collaborative model for knowledge translation between research and practice in clinical settings. *Research in Nursing & Health, 31,* 130–140.

Boyer, E. (1990). *Scholarship reconsidered: Priorities for the American professoriate.* Princeton, NJ: Carnegie Foundation for the Advancement of Teaching.

Cronenwett, L. (2010, January). *Quality and safety implications for doctoral programs in nursing.* Paper presented at the AACN Doctoral Education Conference, Captiva Island, FL.

Cronenwett, L., Sherwood, G., Pohl, J., Barnsteiner, J., Moore, S., Sullivan, D., et al. (2009). Quality and safety education for advanced nursing practice. *Nursing Outlook, 57,* 338–348.

Dracup, K., Cronenwett, L., Meleis, A. I., & Benner, P. E. (2005). Reflections on the doctorate of nursing practice. *Nursing Outlook, 3,* 177–182.

Ellis, R. (1969). Practitioner as theorist. *American Journal of Nursing, 69,* 1434–1438.

Estabrooks, C. A., Thompson, D. S., Lovely, J. E., & Hofmeyer, A. (2006). A guide to knowledge translation theory. *Journal of Continuing Education in the Health Professions, 26*(1), 25–36.

Freshwater, D. (2003). Understanding and implementing clinical nursing research. *Proceedings of the 2003 ICN Biennial Conference, Switzerland.* Retrieved June 13, 2009 from http://www1.icn.ch/48751_4th_proof.pdf

Graham, I. D., Logan, J., Harrison, M. B., Straus, S. E., Tetroe, J., Caswell, W., et al. (2006). Lost in knowledge translation: Time for a map? *Journal of Continuing Education in the Health Professions, 26,* 13–24.

Graham, I. D., & Tetroe, J. (2007). Whither knowledge translation. *Nursing Research, 56*(4S), S86–S88.

Holloway, I., & Wheeler, S. (2002). *Qualitative research in nursing.* Oxford: Blackwell Science.

Horsely, J. A., Crane, J., & Bingle, J. (1978). Research utilization as an organizational process. *Journal of Nursing Administration, 8*(7), 4–6.

Institute of Medicine. (2003). *Health professions education: A bridge to quality.* Washington, DC: National Academies Press.

Institute of Medicine. (2001). *Crossing the quality chasm: A new health system for the 21st century.* Washington, DC: National Academies Press.

Jarvis, P. (2000). The practitioner-researcher in nursing. *Nurse Education Today, 20,* 30–35.

Kirkman, S., Thompson, D. R., Watson, R., & Stewart, S. (2007). Are all doctorates equal or are some "more equal than others"? An examination of which ones should be offered by schools of nursing. *Nurse Education in Practice, 7,* 61–66.

Marion, L., Viens, D., O'Sullivan, A. L., Crabtree, K., Fontana, S., & Price, M. M. (2003). The practice doctorate in nursing: Future or fringe. Topics in Advanced Practice Nursing eJournal. Retrieved January 6, 2010 from http://www.medscape.com/viewarticle/453247

Melnyk, B. M., & Fineout-Overholt, E. (2005). *Evidence-based practice in nursing & healthcare: A guide to best practice.* Philadelphia, PA: Lippincott Williams & Wilkins.

Merriam-Webster Online. (2010). Retrieved April 3, 2010 from http://www.merriam-webster.com/

Newhouse, R., Dearholt, S., Poe, S., Pugh, L., & White, K. (2007). *Johns Hopkins nursing evidence-based practice—Model and guidelines.* Indianapolis, IN: Sigma Theta Tau.

Nonaka, I., Toyama, R., & Konna, N. (2000). SECI, B*a* and leadership: A unified model of dynamic knowledge creation. *Long Range Planning, 33,* 5–34.

Patzek, M. J. (2010). Understanding the DNP degree. *American Nurse Today, 5*(5), 49–50.

Pepper, G. (2010). Bridges on the River Why. *Communicating Nursing Research, 43,* 54.

Ragland, B. (2006). Positioning the practitioner-researcher. *Action Research, 4*(2), 165–182.

Reed, P. G. (2008). Practitioner as theorist: A reprise. *Nursing Science Quarterly, 21*(4), 315–321.

Rolfe, G. (1998). The theory-practice gap in nursing: From research-based practice to practice-based research. *Journal of Advanced Nursing, 28*(3), 672–679.

Rolfe, G., & Davies, R. (2009). Second generation professional doctorates in nursing. *International Journal of Nursing Studies, 46,* 1265–1273.

Rosswurm, M. A., & Larrabee, J. H. (1999). A model for change to evidence-based practice. *Image: Journal of Nursing Scholarship, 31*(4), 317–322.

Sackett, D., Rosenberg, W., Gray, J., & Richardson, W. (1996). Evidence based medicine: What it is and what it is not. *British Medical Journal, 312,* 71–72.

Shulman, L. S., Golde, C. M., Bueschel, A. C., & Garabedian, K. J. (2006). Reclaiming education's doctorates: A critique and a proposal. *Educational Researcher, 35*(3), 25–32.

Smith, M., & McCarthy, M. P. (2010). Disciplinary knowledge in nursing education: Going beyond the blueprints. *Nursing Outlook, 58,* 44–51.

Stephan, W. (2006). Bridging the researcher-practitioner divide in intergroup relations. *Journal of Social Issues, 62*(63), 597–605.

Stetler, C. (1994). Refinement of the Stetler/Marram model for application of research findings to practice. *Nursing Outlook, 42,* 15–25.

Stevens, K. R. (2004). *ACE star model of EBP: Knowledge transformation.* San Antonio, TX: The University of Texas Health Science Center at San Antonio. Retrieved from http://www.acestar.uthscsa.edu

Stevens, K. R., & Staley, J. M. (2006). The Quality Chasm reports, evidence-based practice, and nursing's response to improve healthcare. *Nursing Outlook, 54,* 94–101.

Straus, S. E., Graham, I. D., & Mazmanian, P. E. (2006). Knowledge translation: resolving the confusion. *The Journal of Continuing Education in the Health Professions, 26*(1), 3–4.

Titler, M. G., Kleiber, C., Steelman, V., Rakel, B., Budreau, G., Everett, L. O., et al. (2001). The Iowa model of evidence-based practice to promote quality care. *Critical Care Nursing Clinics of North America, 13*(4), 497–509.

Vincent, D., Johnson, C., Velasquez, D., & Rigney, T. (2010). DNP as "practitioner-researcher": Closing the gap between research and practice. *The American Journal for Nurse Practitioners, 14*(11/12), 24–28.

Whall, A. L. (2005). "Lest we forget": An issue concerning the doctorate of nursing practice (DNP). *Nursing Outlook, 53,* 1.

Woolf, S. H. (2006). The meaning of translational research and why it matters. *Journal of the American Medical Association, 299*(2), 211–213.

Interlude I

The Mandala and Discovering Nursing Worldviews

Nelma B. Crawford Shearer

*A*dvanced practice, doctorally prepared nurses play a significant role in advancing the production of nursing knowledge. They have not only clinical expertise but also a repertoire of patient-practice experiences that serve as a source in developing knowledge, particularly nursing theory. While clinical practice "is the field for knowledge development" (Arslanian-Engoren, Hicks, Whall, & Algase, 2005, p. 317), coursework helps students clarify philosophical perspectives about nursing that are useful in developing one's skills in knowledge production. "Practice is not a 'stand alone' phenomenon" but is an outcome of philosophical beliefs and values (Whall, 2005, p. 1). What is often neglected in theory development to guide interventions is the conceptual work to clarify the nurse's philosophical views and beliefs and concepts of interest that feed the synergy for knowledge between practice and theoretical thinking.

Given the fact that our philosophic views pervade our practice and research, whether we are fully aware of it or not, it is advantageous to take a few moments to consider just what your philosophic views about relevant concepts like health, human beings, environment, and nursing *are*. This can be done by exploring nursing worldviews. Clarifying your own worldview is one of the first steps in developing as a scholar and contributor to nursing knowledge. Your philosophic views are a pathway to inform ethical practice and to stimulate your conceptual ideas. In this *Interlude*, I present a strategy to help you learn about and articulate philosophical views underlying your nursing activities in practice, education, and research.

Nurses engage in what I call *theorizing on their feet* when they integrate theoretical thinking with their practice experiences. This happens more than you may realize. However, historically and still now, theory and practice are regarded as two separate processes. The literature is replete with examples of this. And sometimes it seems that my students have bought into this idea, with emails from them like, "I'm spending more time on this class than any other class. Theory is important to nursing, but I think that I need to spend more time on health assessment and pathophysiology." Nevertheless, I am pleased that students challenge the importance of philosophy and theory in nursing. So to meet this challenge, I developed a teaching strategy to take my students on a journey designed to engage them in theoretical thinking, specifically to clarify their philosophical perspectives about nursing as they look through and perhaps even refocus their practice lens.

LET THE JOURNEY BEGIN

As with all journeys, learning to "theorize on your feet" begins with foundational steps. One way to begin is with a theory class assignment to help you describe and ponder the role of nursing science (Barrett, 2002) or debate the purpose of nursing theory in practice (Cody, 2003). These kinds of readings introduce you to elements that comprise nursing's structure of knowledge including worldviews, the nursing metaparadigm, and theories. The readings are also useful in exploring the relationships among abstract terms like *science, practice, research,* and *theory.* But perhaps the most important assignment, once you have knowledge of what some of the experts say about nursing science and theory, is to consider your *own* expertise and to reflect on the ideas *you* cherish in nursing.

Using ideas from the readings and reflections on practice, I invite students to discuss a few deceptively simple questions drawn from the readings and posted on our online discussion board: "What is the focus of our discipline?" "When you walk into your patient's room, what do you first observe and assess?" "Why?" With a little coaching, students notice that their responses to the first question may reflect our nursing metaparadigm concepts: health, person–environment, nursing practice. Or students may discover other key concepts not yet considered as part of the nursing metaparadigm. Responses to the second question often address technology and the machines hooked up to the patient. During the online discussion, one doctoral student began to question her perception of the patient for whom she most recently provided care. "As I look back on the past few weeks," she reflected,

> I am trying to remember if I viewed my patient and/or their family as a whole, instead of their parts. I think it's easy to get caught up in taking care of a patient from a physiological perspective and not remembering the person has thoughts, feelings, and is part of a family.

These discussions of the readings—as informed by students' practice experiences—serve as a catalyst to spark creativity in thinking theoretically as well as philosophically—that is, to think about their interest area for inquiry and then to delve deeper into the *why* behind their interests or what worldviews influence their thinking.

WORLDVIEWS IN NURSING

A worldview or paradigm reflects the discipline as a whole and the subject matter addressed by the discipline. A worldview seeks to answer two types of philosophical issues: views of reality (ontology) and views of knowledge (epistemology) (Arslanian-Engoren et al., 2005).

Several philosophical perspectives have been offered by nursing scholars. Newman, Sime, and Corcoran-Perry (1991) offer three perspectives on nursing theory and the development of practice knowledge: the particulate-deterministic, the interactive-integrative, and the unitary-transformative. From an analysis of these and other worldviews, Fawcett (1993) arrived at the worldviews of reaction, reciprocal-interaction, and simultaneous action.

A nurse practicing from the *particulate-deterministic or reaction* perspective views phenomena as reducible, definable properties that are orderly and predictably connected to one another. Change is viewed as something that can be controlled. Human beings are viewed as bio-psycho-social-spiritual beings. The metaphor for human beings is the "machine" (Reed, 1995).

The *interactive-integrative* or *reciprocal-interaction* perspective presents phenomena as having multiple interrelated parts and change as a function of multiple factors and probabilistic relationships (Fawcett, 1993; Newman et al., 1991). Human beings are viewed as holistic, with parts understood within the context of the whole. Human beings are active, acting upon a passive environment. The biologic organism is the metaphor for human beings (Reed, 1995).

From the *unitary-transformative* or *simultaneous-action* perspective, the nurse views phenomena as unitary, self-organizing, identified by pattern, and in process with the environment (Fawcett, 1993; Newman et al., 1991). Change in human beings and their environment is ongoing and unpredictable. The historical event (with the person as embedded in ongoing change and a historical context) is the metaphor for human beings (Reed, 1995).

PHILOSOPHICAL VIEW

Perhaps because of their perceived lack of familiarity with the theory dimension of their science, doctoral nursing students are eager to find ways to bring conceptual ideas, including their own philosophic views, to the forefront of their practice. They know that theory is a source of knowledge for improving patient care while optimizing patient health. However, theory and theorizing may provide little meaning until theory is personalized. So, I designed a learning experience, involving a mandala to help students begin to personalize the theory process, beginning with their own broad philosophical ideas.

I recalled Dr. Margaret Newman presenting her theory "Health as Expanding Consciousness" in picture form. During her presentation and the dialogue that followed, participants shared ideas and techniques they used to express their various philosophical perspectives. One example highlighted the drawing of a mandala. When used in a course, I thought perhaps this drawing activity could help students elucidate new meanings and organize their ideas as they grappled with nursing theory and knowledge production, particularly as related to their practice experiences. It was time to refocus my lens! I endeavored to expand my more traditional approach of teaching nursing theory through reading and discussion activities, to an approach that highlighted and captured students' creative processes.

ROLE OF THE MANDALA IN EXPRESSING A WORLDVIEW

The word *mandala* comes from the classical Indian language of Sanskrit and means "circle" (The Mandala Project, n.d.). The circular shape signifies wholeness and can be viewed as an organizing framework with a unifying center. Mandalas contain symbols and patterns regarding all aspects of life and nature, such as in the earth and the sun, a flower, or a snowflake. The mandala is also used to depict a circle of life, including a community of friends and family. The mandala pattern is visible in certain cultures, religious traditions as well as in architecture. For example, American Indians have used a circular shape to create the medicine wheel, whereas religious groups create circles or labyrinths for meditation and architects design structures built around a center.

Since a mandala contains symbols and patterns that are meaningful to you, creating your own mandala may increase awareness of and thinking about your values and beliefs, that is, your philosophical views, as they may influence your practice and research. A self-exploration as framed within a mandala provides an opportunity to begin thinking about your choices and beliefs as they play out in your perspectives and activities in nursing. In addition, creating a mandala by focusing on nursing's four metaparadigm concepts may sensitize you to values and beliefs that are blended unconsciously into your everyday practice.

SELF-EXPLORATION

To initiate your self-exploration, put this book down for a moment and reflect on your practice experiences and readings on theory and research literature. Think of strategies you might use to relax and open up to new ideas. For example, enjoy a walk, sit outside and relish the cool breeze of the early morning or late afternoon, take a swim, find a quiet place inside or outside under a tree, or listen to some music. Next, view the world as a mandala: a circle with a unifying center. Incorporate visual cues from nature with your nursing practice experiences and begin to create a mandala of nursing's metaparadigm: person, environment, health, and nurse.

Questions to guide you in this reflection are as follows: "What is the focal point of my mental picture?" "Is it the patient, nurse, health, environment or something else?" From there, draw the picture that is in your mind on a piece of paper or go to your computer and recreate your mental picture. If you are having trouble creating your picture, let the idea of a mandala or circle assist you in turning your visualization into a picture. Look at your drawing and think about your practice; what is the organizing framework and unifying center? Is person, nurse, health, or environment at the center of your practice? Step back and reflect on your drawing as you have produced a creative vision of your everyday practice. "How do you define or characterize these broad concepts?" Now think about your worldview or your philosophical perspective of nursing. "Do you view people as machines, a biologic organism, or from a developmental, historical perspective?" Think about your practice experiences: "What is the unifying center of your practice experiences?"

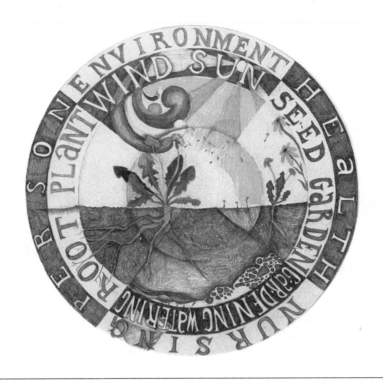

FIGURE 3.1

Mandala and Description by Timothy Kruth. Reprinted with permission by Timothy Kruth.

Description of Mandala (Figure 3.1): Person (composed of roots and plant). I represented the *person* with a plant. It is divided in two specific ways, particularly in its interaction with the environment (the plant portion) and the nursing (the root portion). Together they make up one full person (dandelion) and neither can exist without the other. I chose a dandelion as they are highly resilient, show distinct stages, and are common throughout the world. The plant is large in size to acknowledge the plant itself and its physical entity but also skewed to one side to equally incorporate the environmental, health, and nursing aspects of the individual, acknowledging that those factors highly influence the plant's overall health. Environment (composed of wind and sun). The environment composes the *external forces* which both benefit and harm the life cycle. Both the wind and the sun represent necessary factors to allow growth and energy (sun providing energy), and progression (wind blowing seeds) in life. Health (composed of seed and garden). This aspect of the metaparadigm incorporates the plant's *life progression and purpose for existence*. This includes the interpretations of the physical, cultural, and spiritual aspects of life. The progression of the plant (seed) signifies the plant's autonomy as only a healthy plant that exists harmoniously with the other three major categories will propagate and flourish amidst a community (garden). This category further includes the person's views on normal health progression and life after death. Nursing (composed of watering and gardening). This portion of the represented metaparadigm related the external aspects of natural watering and gardening and the spiritual/God influence on our lives. It is an action performed by any *intentional* external autonomous presence in order to benefit the health of the person. In this category, both the human and spiritual forces necessary and benefiting survival exist. Nursing involves caring, skill, and particular knowledge in taking care of the plant and its needs.

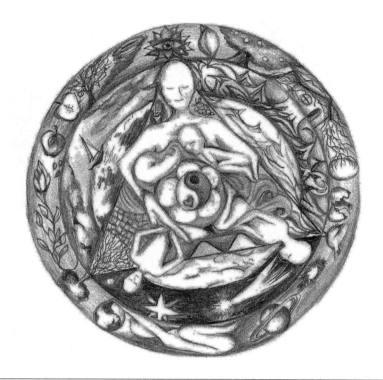

FIGURE 3.2

Mandala and Description by Lisa Green. Reprinted with permission by Lisa Green.

Description of Mandala (Figure 3.2): Person-singular soul in universe, living spirit researching for soul enrichment through experience in life, conception, seed, egg, growth, and death complete the life circle of continuing human evolvement. Health-obtained from harmony in living on the earth and dreaming of the universe, progression obtained with well being in existence. Seek pathway for continued well being in existence. Environment-sun is source of energy for creation of life, earth is provider of life energy with collaboration of sun's energy and earth is mother for shelter and sustenance, the capsule of life suspended in the universe of unknowns. Nursing-facilitates pathway creation for harmony in health and environment for person, to achieve balance in earthly existence, support dream of universe and place in existence by promotion of love through caring.

ARTICULATING A WORLDVIEW AS A LINK TO PRACTICE

Based on your worldview, the center of the drawing may consist of anything from stick figures to an elaborate drawing with the focal point of a patient, nurse, environment, or health. Regardless of the focal point, think about the center of your drawing and why you chose this as your focal point in relationship to worldviews in nursing.

Next, consider which nursing worldview your mandala most portrays. Do you perceive the patient and practice from the *particulate-deterministic* or *reaction* perspective worldview in which human beings are viewed as machines and health is viewed as a consequence of a single event? That is, do you emphasize a cause–effect relationship in which the patient returns to a state of equilibrium, with balance as the health goal (Reed, 1995). If this worldview is congruent with your perspective, you may view your role as developing a care plan for the patient that focuses on reducing personal risk for disease and death.

If your worldview is more in line with the *interactive-integrative* or reciprocal-interaction perspective, you perceive a human being as a living biological open system (Reed, 1995). Health and illness occur simultaneously within the human–environment relationship. In your practice, you center your attention on optimizing the patient's health while focusing on the patient rather than his or her environment.

The *unitary-transformative* or *simultaneous-action* worldview proposes that there are many ways of viewing and explaining health and the patient. If this worldview appears to be congruent with your perspective as reflected in your mandala, you may believe that health and illness occur simultaneously within the human–environment process and are not viewed as separate events. Changes in health occur through an interactive relationship with the environment that are ongoing and irreversible, innovative, and developmental (Reed, 1995). You perceive the patient as interacting with the environment and recognize health as embedded in a context that changes from moment to moment. When practicing from this worldview, you focus on the patient as well as their family and environment to optimize their well-being.

LET THE JOURNEY CONTINUE

Whether you realize it or not, you have begun the process of philosophic inquiry by clarifying some of your own beliefs and definitions about concepts basic to nursing. This in turn provides a personal foundation for making some of the choices you will face as a practitioner and knowledge-builder of nursing. Now, turn to Chapter 1 and revisit the section that highlights the philosophy of nursing path. Review Reed's philosophic inquiry questions intended to inspire your scientific inquiry in practice and research by asking yourself "What is nursing?" "What are the elements of a human being that nursing should attend to?" "How do I define health, and is it ethical to apply my definition to patients?" These questions may never go away, and you may revisit them again and again as you pursue a scholarly career in nursing.

Regardless of where the process begins, self-exploration and articulating a worldview through a mandala is intended to enhance understanding of your own philosophy about human beings, health, nursing, and the environment—nursing's metaparadigm. In addition, your descriptions of the metaparadigm concepts provide a framework for recognizing your worldview of nursing and either refocusing or confirming your practice lens. Let the journey that began with self-exploration and culminated in the recognition of your worldview continue as you develop into a scholar and contributor to nursing knowledge.

QUESTIONS FOR REFLECTION

1. Based on your drawing, what worldview or philosophic views seem congruent with your practice?
2. How has this chapter helped you refocus your practice lens?
3. Which of the mandalas presented here do you prefer and why, in terms of the philosophic views it conveys to you?
4. What role could recognizing your worldview play in your development as a scholar and contributor to nursing knowledge?

———————

REFERENCES

Arslanian-Engoren, C., Hicks, F. D., Whall, A. L., & Algase, D. L. (2005). An ontological view of advanced practice nursing. *Research and Theory for Nursing Practice, 19*, 315–322.

Barrett, E. A. M. (2002). What is nursing science? *Nursing Science Quarterly, 15*(1), 51–60.

Cody, W. K. (2003). Nursing theory as a guide to practice. *Nursing Science Quarterly, 16*, 225–231.

Fawcett, J. (1993). For a plethora of paradigms to parsimony in worldviews. *Nursing Science Quarterly, 6*(3), 56–59.

The Mandala Project. (n.d.). Retrieved May 20, 2010, from http://www.mandalaproject.org/what/index.html

Newman, M. A., Sime, A. M., & Corcoran-Perry, S. A. (1991). The focus of the discipline of nursing. *Advances in Nursing Science, 14*(1), 1–6.

Reed, P. G. (1995). A treatise on nursing knowledge development for the 21st century: Beyond postmodernism. *Advances in Nursing Science, 17*(3), 70–84.

Whall, A. L. (2005). "Lest we forget": An issue concerning the doctorate of nursing practice (DNP). *Nursing Outlook, 53*(1), 1.

Practitioner-Centered Research: Nursing Praxis and the Science of the Unique

Gary Rolfe

Where is the wisdom we have lost in knowledge?
Where is the knowledge we have lost in information?
   T.S. Eliot, 1934/1940, First Chorus from "The Rock"

It is perhaps disingenuous of me to begin a chapter on practitioner research in nursing practice with this particular quote from T.S. Eliot, since he was bemoaning the very "endless cycle of idea and action, endless invention, endless experiment" (Eliot, 1934/1940) that I intend to advocate. When Eliot used the word *wisdom*, he was referring to the outcome of a process of silent internal contemplation which he identified as prayer, but which, in the secular world of nursing practice, we might describe as reflection-on-action (Schön, 1983), the thoughtful contemplation of prior practice. However, this chapter is concerned with another form of wisdom which arises from another form of reflection; that is, with the clinical wisdom or wise action that results from Schön's (1983) reflection-*in*-action or on-the-spot experimenting.

I intend to use Eliot's ascending hierarchy of information, knowledge, and wisdom as a framework for my critique of the current paradigm of nursing research and evidence-based practice and my subsequent exploration of nursing praxis, the integration of research and practice in the clinical setting. I will suggest in particular that the recent move toward evidence-based practice as the underpinning rationale for clinical nursing has led to an abandonment of the search for wisdom, and even for knowledge and theory, in favor of the accumulation of information about the comparative effectiveness and efficiency of different nursing interventions.

Eliot was right to point out that the descent from wisdom to information entails a loss. However, there is a real danger for nursing that the loss is not recognized and that practitioners act in the mistaken belief that wise actions can be reconstituted from information that has had all of the rich, contextual personal knowledge stripped from it. As educationalist Lawrence Stenhouse (1978) warned,

Without understanding why one course of action is better than another, we could prove by statistical treatment that it is. The vision is an enticing one: it suggests that we may make wise judgments without understanding what we are doing. (p. 28)

The purpose of this chapter is to argue that the social and medical research paradigms adopted by the academic discipline of nursing are no longer fit for purpose in the 21st century and to propose that we consider in their place a science of the unique person underpinned by praxis, the coming together of research and practice in a single, seamless act.

ACADEMIC NURSING AND THE RISE OF NURSING THEORY

As with many emerging professions, the advent of modern nursing in the mid-19th century was preceded by many years before its acceptance as a full academic discipline. The date and manner of the entry of nursing into the academy is open to dispute but might for convenience be taken as 1923 when Yale opened the first independent university-based school for the education of nurses. However, if we measure the maturity of an academic discipline by the widespread award of master's and doctoral degrees, then the discipline of nursing only came of age in the 1970s in the United States (Kalisch & Kalisch, 1995) and even later in other parts of the world.

Prior to its entry into the academy, the theoretical underpinning of the practice of nursing consisted predominantly of Nightingale's twin pillars of public health and compassionate caring (Nightingale, 1860). However, many of the early master's programs in nursing admitted graduates in disciplines other than nursing, culminating in a generation of nurse academics who brought with them a range of theories and methods from other disciplines, mostly in the social sciences. This in turn led to a broadening out of theoretical perspectives and a particular emphasis on social science research paradigms as the primary means of conceptualizing and generating nursing knowledge. More recently, the evidence-based practice movement has heralded a move away from grand and middle-range theory generation and testing in nursing toward a more pragmatic and eclectic approach in which nursing practice is shaped and directed predominantly according to the findings of quantitative evaluation studies and randomized trials.

The term *nursing research* is therefore nowadays applied to two separate and in many ways distinct fields of scholarly activity. On one hand, many nurse researchers continue to employ the methods and methodologies of the social sciences, particularly from sociology and anthropology, to develop, test, and modify nursing theory. On the other hand, a small but growing group of researchers are using the experimental and quasi-experimental methodologies derived from medicine and (as we shall see) agriculture to test the effectiveness and efficacy of specific nursing interventions in clinical trials. These two groups of nurse researchers often come into conflict, with the social scientists claiming that the experimentalists have no regard for theory and the traditions of nursing, and the experimentalists claiming that the social scientists are advocating practice that is not based on robust and rigorous scientific evidence.

While the methods and methodologies of each camp have their uses and have undoubtedly made valuable contributions to the practice of nursing, I will suggest in this chapter that neither of them is sufficiently grounded in nursing practice to make the claim to be fully "nursing research." In particular, I will argue that whereas the methods and methodologies of social research and clinical trials have evolved to meet the needs of the social sciences and medicine, respectively, nursing practice has a very different agenda and focus from either of these disciplines and requires a very different approach to the generation and application of knowledge. Indeed, I will suggest that a discipline such as nursing, whose focus and goals revolve around practice, requires a different understanding not only of how knowledge should be generated but also of what knowledge *is*. This in turn implies a radical reconceptualization of what it means to be an academic discipline (and, on a personal level, what it means to be an academic) in a practice-based profession. This challenge is set out clearly by Donald Schön (1983) in his investigation into the demands of "professional education," that is, education for practice:

> We are in need of inquiry into an epistemology of practice. What is the kind of knowing in which competent practitioners engage? How is professional knowing like and unlike the kinds of knowledge presented in academic textbooks, scientific papers, and learned journals? In what sense, if any, is there intellectual rigor in professional practice? (p. viii)

This chapter will attempt to address some of Schön's (1983) questions and will outline a new epistemology of nursing that pays attention, in Schön's words, to the kind of knowing in which competent practitioners engage. This task includes not only an examination of what practitioners need to know but also of the ways in which that knowledge is constructed and what, if anything, should count as intellectual rigor in a discipline for which the focus of inquiry is ultimately the development of practice rather than theory. In short, this chapter will propose and explore the argument that most of the research methods and methodologies currently considered to be central to the discipline of nursing are, in fact, *fundamentally* unsuitable and ill-equipped to generate the kinds of knowledge that nurses require for practice in the 21st century.

NURSING AND THE SOCIAL SCIENCES

A brief scan through the contents pages of any of the major nursing research textbooks from the past 30 years or so will confirm that nursing research has become intimately associated with the methodologies and methods of the social sciences, particularly with sociology and anthropology. This has been due in part to the generally accepted definition of nursing as a social activity and in part to a significant number of prominent and influential nurse academics having had a prior grounding in various social science disciplines and their respective research methods and methodologies. I will therefore begin with a discussion of the aims of social research and an exploration of how they differ from the requirements of nursing practice.

It is widely accepted by social scientists that the primary and perhaps sole purpose of social research is to generate, test, and inform social knowledge and theory, and it has usually been considered sufficient merely to change the word *social* to *nursing* to produce a paradigm for nursing research. I will suggest that this uncritical embracing of the methodologies of social research into nursing is problematic in a number of ways. First, it immediately sets out the expectation that nursing and the social sciences should share similar aims, methods, and epistemologies and, indeed, that nursing *is* a social science. Second, it assumes that the primary function and purpose of nursing research should be to produce nursing knowledge. Third, it implies that research can only inform practice through the medium of knowledge and theory and thus locates practice at least one degree removed from research. Fourth, and following on from this assumption, it suggests that the kinds of knowledge generated by the social science research methods and methodologies can be applied in a more or less direct and unproblematic way to nursing practice.

The relationship outlined above between research on one hand and knowledge and theory on the other has been accepted more or less uncritically in nursing and has subsequently become so entrenched as to be almost axiomatic. To suggest that the purpose of nursing research might be *something other* than to produce or test nursing knowledge and (to a lesser extent) nursing theory is generally considered misguided at best and heretical at worst. Thus, Polit and Beck (2004) define nursing research as "systematic inquiry designed to develop *knowledge* about issues of importance to the nursing profession" and clinical nursing research as "designed to generate *knowledge* to guide nursing practice and to improve the health and quality of life of nurses' clients" (p. 3, italics added). The essence of these definitions is repeated throughout the literature, and it is widely accepted that the purpose of nursing research is predominantly to generate knowledge which can be employed by nurses to enhance their practice.

Implicit in this conception of nursing research is a one-way hierarchical relationship in which research leads to improved knowledge and knowledge leads to improved practice. This in turn implies a similar one-way hierarchical relationship between researchers and practitioners, where nurses are expected to base their practice primarily on the work of academics who are often no longer (or, indeed, may never have been) clinically active. As Greenwood (1966) pointed out nearly half a century ago:

> In the evolution of every profession there emerges the researcher-theoretician whose role is that of scientific investigation and theoretical systematization. In technological professions, a division of labor thereby evolves between the theory-oriented and the practice-oriented person. (p. 12)

Priyjmachuk (1996) added that, in the discipline of nursing, "it is the theories of the pure scientists that dictate the actions of those in practice," and "though a relationship between theory and practice appears to exist, it seems somewhat unidirectional in nature" (p. 680). Schön (1983) referred to this unidirectional flow of knowledge from research to practice in the professions as technical rationality.

While such a hierarchical relationship between research and practice and between researchers and practitioners might be appropriate in the social science disciplines, it is far less straightforward when the social science research methodologies are applied to practice disciplines such as nursing, for which they were never originally intended.

The main difficulty with applying the findings from social research methodologies to the practice of nursing becomes immediately apparent when we consider the purpose for which social research was originally developed. Sociology has been defined in simple terms as "the scientific study of human life, social groups, whole societies and the human world" (Giddens, 2009, p. 3).

The original purpose of social research was to understand and predict the *collective behavior* of social groups and societies to inform practical and policy decisions about social institutions and relationships. Even in social science disciplines such as anthropology, where the focus is often on small and sometimes idiosyncratic groups and organizations, the aim is usually to produce an objective and scientific account which allows us to make inferences to human behavior *in general*. Thus

> The culture is turned into an object available for study…[and] it is possible to construct an account of the culture under investigation that captures it as external to, and independent of, the researcher; in other words, as a natural phenomenon. (Hammersley & Atkinson, 1983, p. 8)

The implications of this description are first that anthropology can be safely regarded as an objective science and second that it is akin to the natural sciences insofar as culture is presented as a widespread and naturally occurring phenomenon. These twin assumptions allowed the founding mothers and fathers of cultural anthropology to make the claim that it enabled "advanced" societies to understand the history of their own social development by studying cultures that are operating at a supposedly more "primitive" level, in much the same way that palaeontologists can trace biological development by studying primitive organisms.

Even the more ideographic social research methodologies such as phenomenology can be seen to be underpinned by realist and/or positivist assumptions about essence and generalizability. Thus

> Phenomenological researchers ask: What is the *essence* of this phenomenon as experienced by these people and what does it *mean*? Phenomenologists assume there is an essence—an essential invariant structure—that can be understood, in much the same way that ethnographers assume that cultures exist. Phenomenologists investigate subjective phenomena in the belief that critical *truths about reality* are grounded in people's lived experiences. (Polit & Beck, 2006, p. 219, italics added)

The stated purpose of phenomenology, at least as it is presented here, is to uncover truths about reality through a process of "bracket[ing] out the world and any presuppositions in an effort to confront the data in pure form" (Polit & Beck, 2006, p. 220). Although phenomenologists typically work with small samples, the aim is to make universal statements about essential truths based on common categories of "lived experiences."

It is fair to say, then, that social science is a macroscience that attempts to describe, measure, and predict attitudes and behaviors at the level of large groups or whole societies. The main purpose of social research is to categorize these attitudes, feelings, and behaviors to make inductive generalizations from a representative sample to a larger group, and the various social research methods and methodologies have been designed and developed largely with that purpose in mind.

When the research methods and methodologies of the social sciences were first introduced into the academic discipline of nursing in the 1960s and 1970s, it could be argued that they offered an appropriate paradigm for the profession. At that time, nursing care was usually organized and delivered in a task-centered way with a focus on finding the most efficient and effective means of providing routine and standardized care to large numbers of patients (Anderson, 1973). As the Royal College of Nursing (RCN) in the United Kingdom pointed out at the time,

> To see nursing as a one-to-one relationship, even when that relationship is between the individual nurse and the individual patient, is to narrow down the concept of the nurse's role. The individual must be seen as a member of a group, and the group within the context of society. (RCN, 1971)

Research methods that provided statistical information about the general effectiveness of different approaches to various nursing tasks at the level of the group or society were therefore of great benefit in streamlining ward routines at a time when the completion of tasks often provided more satisfaction to nurses than patient-oriented goals (McLean, 1973).

It could be argued, however, that the academic discipline of nursing has failed to keep pace with subsequent changes to nursing practice. Since the introduction of the social science paradigm for the production and testing of nursing knowledge and theory, the focus of practice has shifted from the group to the individual. We can see this shift in the most recent definition of nursing from the RCN, which refers to caring for "*individuals* of all ages, families and communities, throughout the entire life span" and adds that

> the specific domain of nursing is people's *unique responses* to and experience of health, illness, frailty, disability and health related life events in whatever environment or circumstances they find themselves. (RCN, 2010, italics added)

This represents a complete *volte-face* for the RCN from their earlier definition of nursing as a social activity and is echoed by the International Council for Nurses (ICN) in their statement that "nursing encompasses autonomous and collaborative care of *individuals* of all ages, families, groups and communities, sick or well and in all settings" (ICN, 2010, italics added).

It would seem, then, that academic nursing has not kept pace with the fundamental changes in the focus of practice. Although social research methods and methodologies might be appropriate for informing nursing policy and decisions at a macro level, they were never intended to tell us anything about what happens at the micro level of the unique therapeutic encounter between unique individuals in a unique setting at a unique moment in time. For this purpose, as we might expect, what is required is not a science of society informed by objective and generalizable research methodologies but *a science of the unique,* informed by methods and methodologies designed to provide individualized and contextualized knowledge that arises from and relates directly back to practice (Rolfe, 2006a; Rolfe & Gardner, 2005).

NURSING AND EVIDENCE-BASED PRACTICE

Despite the argument for a more individualized approach, recent trends in nursing research appear to be moving in the very opposite direction. Nursing has for many years aspired to be recognized as a research-based profession, and as we have seen, this has generally been interpreted and understood in terms of the qualitative and quantitative methods and methodologies of the social science research paradigms. However, the past decade has increasingly witnessed a shift away from *research*-based practice toward *evidence*-based practice. On one level, this shift has been hardly noticeable, since many practitioners and some academics regard the two terms as more or less synonymous, often using the words *research* and *evidence* interchangeably. A closer examination of the tenets of evidence-based practice (EBP), however, reveals a clear bias toward evidence from experimental and quasi-experimental research studies and a subsequent shift from the social science research paradigms to the paradigms of medicine and agriculture.

Many advocates of EBP argue for a hierarchy in which the quality of the evidence is rated solely according to its method of production, and a number of hierarchies of evidence have been published over the past decade, all of which place evidence from randomized controlled trials (RCTs), and preferably evidence from systematic reviews of *several* RCTs, at the top. As Morton and Morton (2003) assert, "Evidence comes in many forms and varies in quality. Within research, there is a recognized hierarchy of reliability that can be used as a guide when considering the effectiveness of evidence." (http://www.ebnp.co.uk/The%20Hierarchy%20of%20 Evidence.htm) Their own hierarchy, in keeping with most others, places evidence from systematic reviews and RCTs at the top and descriptive studies and evidence from experience at the bottom.

The EBP movement clearly plays down the findings from nonexperimental social research, which is considered to be a lowly form of evidence and is only acceptable if it derives from more than one study by more than one research group. Although Polit and Beck (2008) suggest hopefully that "in the current evidence-based environment, there is likely to be an increase in small, localized research designed to solve immediate problems" (p. 10), such studies are unlikely to meet the strict criteria outlined above. What is more likely, and is in fact already happening in the United Kingdom, is that research is becoming industrialized with large multidisciplinary teams conducting multimillion dollar production-line research projects with a division of labor in which each researcher has responsibility for only a small part of the research process and rarely gets an overview of the entire project. Nursing research is therefore becoming further removed from everyday practice and practitioners as small, individualized, and unfunded projects are being diminished in impact and importance.

However, the shift from research-based practice to evidence-based practice could be seen as far more dangerous and insidious than simply a scaling-up of research activity. I have already suggested that the social science research paradigms have located the focus of nursing research in the domain of knowledge and theory-testing rather than in practice, which in T.S. Eliot's phrase represents the loss of wisdom at the expense of knowledge. Evidence-based practice, at least in its original and generally understood form, suggests a further shift in the focus of nursing research away from the traditional social science aim of *Verstehen* or understanding toward the scientific testing of nursing and medical interventions to produce "evidence" of their efficacy. The EBP movement has little regard for the building or testing of theory and is concerned primarily with effectiveness and efficiency; it is interested less in developing a coherent body of professional knowledge than in presenting an atheoretical patchwork of "experimentally tested" interventions. In T.S. Eliot's term, this represents the loss of knowledge in favor of information.

CHALLENGES TO THE HIERARCHY OF EVIDENCE

I suggested in the introduction to this chapter that the descent from wisdom to knowledge and to information entails a loss that cannot be retrieved. Wisdom can be reduced to knowledge but knowledge alone cannot be used to reconstitute that wisdom. Similarly, knowledge can be reduced to information, but information alone cannot be used to reconstruct knowledge. From this perspective, the data generated by RCTs might well offer practitioners reliable and valid information about the effectiveness of various nursing interventions, but it cannot provide them with the clinical wisdom necessary to make judicious decisions about the application of that information. Seen from this perspective, the findings from RCTs are of limited use to the practicing nurse; they provide the nurse with general population-level data that might or might not be taken into consideration as background information for clinical decisions, but they do not help in making the on-the-spot clinical judgments demanded of the wise practitioner.

Given that RCTs are located at the apex of most hierarchies of evidence, this is, perhaps, a surprising claim that requires further examination. The randomized controlled trial, which is the foundation of evidence-based practice, is widely acknowledged as having its origins in agricultural research (Fisher, 1935), where it was developed as a means of comparing the effectiveness of pesticides or fertilizers on identical fields of crops. In its original format, then, the outcome measure of the RCT was overall crop yield, and the fate of individual plants was largely irrelevant. The RCT methodology was later applied to medicine, usually to test the efficacy and safety of newly developed drugs. Similarly, the outcome measure was usually taken to be overall clinical improvement or lessening of side effects in the experimental group when compared with a control group.

Clearly, the transition from agriculture to medicine entailed a number of modifications to the methodology. First, of course, medical researchers could not neglect the welfare of the individual; although it did not matter whether individual plants in the experimental group died, so long as there was an increase in overall yield, the same attitude could not be taken with human subjects in a drug trial. Second, refinements such as double blinds had to be introduced in recognition of some fundamental differences between plants and sentient humans. However, the methodology remained essentially the same: A treatment was considered to be more effective if the group of subjects to whom it was administered responded better than the group who received a placebo.

In cases where the treatment intervention is a drug or a medical procedure, the logic of the clinical trial is more or less sound: If a carefully selected and representative sample from a particular population responds to the intervention, then we can say with some statistical level of certainty that the entire population from which the sample was drawn will respond in a similar manner. What the trial does not enable us to do, however, is to make predictions about individual members of the population or about the effectiveness of the treatment in other contexts and settings. In the case of crop treatments or medical drugs, that hardly matters, since the assumption is that all members of the population will respond in much the same way regardless of the social, temporal, or physical context in which the treatment is administered (although, of course, the introduction of the double blind is a tacit acknowledgement of a social or psychological factor in physical responses to medicines). However, I have argued above that clinical nursing practice is composed of a series of personal and unique interventions whose outcome will depend on a large number of social and contextual factors; indeed, that these social and contextual factors are sometimes of greater relevance to the outcome than the treatment itself. For the nurse, then, *information* about the average response to a nursing intervention by the population as a whole will not readily translate into *knowledge* about the idiosyncratic responses of individual patients or into clinical *wisdom* about whether to employ a particular intervention in a particular case with a particular patient in a particular setting at a particular time.

I am arguing that the hierarchy of evidence, with randomized controlled trials at its pinnacle and nonexperimental studies and experiential knowledge at the bottom, does not reflect the important and fundamental differences between the practice of medicine and the practice of nursing. A number of writers have responded to this discrepancy by proposing a new conceptualization of evidence-based *nursing* that takes into account the specific demands of the discipline. For example, Mulhall (1998) argued that "tiptoeing in the wake of the movement for evidence based medicine, we must ensure that evidence based nursing attends to what is important for nursing" (p. 4) and suggested that evidence from qualitative studies should be given equal status to evidence from RCTs. However, while a paradigm of evidence-based *nursing* might replace the RCT with qualitative methodologies at the apex of the hierarchy of evidence, such an approach nevertheless maintains and reinforces the separation between research and practice and between researchers and practitioners.

EBP AND TECHNICAL RATIONALITY

I wish to suggest, however, that the problem for nursing practice is deeper and more complex than simply a dispute over quantitative, qualitative, or (more recently) mixed-method approaches to the generation of research evidence. As I argued earlier, the issue is not so much a question of what kind of research evidence should form the basis of nursing practice but rather the very idea that nursing should be *based* on research evidence at all. Although this might appear to be a somewhat perverse claim, the question of what it means to base practice on research evidence is complex and pivotal to evidence-based practice but has been largely avoided by advocates of the EBP movement.

The original prospectus for evidence-based practice, as set out by the Evidence-Based Medicine Working Group (1992), claimed that "evidence-based medicine de-emphasizes intuition [and] unsystematic clinical experience…and stresses the examination of evidence from clinical research" (p. 2420), specifically the RCT. Little was said about how the evidence was to be implemented, although Sackett, Rosenberg, Gray, Haynes, and Richardson (1996) later added that the practice of evidence-based medicine somehow entailed "integrating individual clinical expertise with the best available external clinical evidence from systematic research" (p. 71).

Precisely how individual clinical expertise and generalizable scientific research findings were to be integrated was never made clear, although Sackett et al. (1996) instructed that the clinical judgments of individual practitioners should always take precedence over research evidence. Presumably, these clinical judgments are based on the very same "unsystematic clinical experience" that the Evidence-Based Medicine Working Group claimed should be "de-emphasized," and it is difficult to conceptualize a model of evidence-based practice in which the evidence from "gold standard" research findings can, at any time, be overthrown by the unsystematic and unscientific judgments of the practitioner. Perhaps for these reasons, advocates of evidence-based approaches have tended to focus almost exclusively on the concept of *evidence* and have neglected to explore the equally important but vague and under theorized notion of what it means to *base* practice on evidence.

When nurse academics first began to explore the possibilities for EBP in nursing, they imported the medical version more or less wholesale, retaining not only the importance of systematic research based on scientific rigor but also the emphasis on the concept of "evidence" and the relative neglect of the second word in the phrase "evidence-based practice." So, for example, French defined EBP in nursing as "the process of systematic identification, rigorous evaluation and the subsequent dissemination and use of the findings of research to influence clinical practice" (French, 1998, p. 47).

While she identified "evidence" as the identification, evaluation, and dissemination of research findings, with the "gold standard" being the randomized controlled trial, little consideration was given to how, in her words, evidence might *influence* clinical practice; that is, to what it means for practice to be *based* on evidence from research. Indeed, the translation of evidence into practice has usually been considered so straightforward as to barely merit a mention.

Although this might perhaps be the case in many medical settings, where evidence-based practice could mean simply the prescription of a drug or treatment regime that a clinical trial has shown to be effective, I have suggested that nursing practice is somewhat more complex and individualized. If evidence-based nursing is to have any authentic practical meaning, our definition of the concept of what might count as best evidence will be secondary to and dependent on what, if anything, it means for nursing practice to be *based* on evidence.

BEYOND TECHNICAL RATIONALITY

We can see that the word *based* acts here as a conjunctive, a word that serves to join the two separate and disparate activities of doing research and doing practice, thereby reinforcing the hierarchy advocated by technical rationality: Research and practice are linked in a causal relationship in which research activity determines evidence and evidence determines nursing practice. Rather than simply replace one research methodology with another at the top of a hierarchy of nursing evidence, I wish to advocate the radical approach of abandoning technical rationality altogether as the dominant paradigm for nursing practice. In other words, I want to propose an approach to doing nursing that is not *based* on evidence from externally conducted research but which integrates the collection and application of evidence into the practice of nursing itself.

If nursing practice is thought of as a series of unique encounters between individuals, then information about what tends to happen *in the average case* will be of limited use in making wise judgments about what to do *in any particular case*. Indeed, it could be argued that the only research findings that will be of any immediate practical use are those that arise from the specific case itself. This suggests that we should value and prioritize research evidence in nursing *not* according to whether it has been generated by the application of a rigorous, objective, controlled, decontextualized, and generalizable "scientific" methodology such as the RCT but by the extent to which it will be of benefit to the specific clinical situation in which the nurse currently finds herself. Generalized macro-level information might be of some limited use in discerning trends and possibilities, but the most important and valuable knowledge required by a nurse who needs to make a wise clinical decision *here and now with this unique individual patient* is the rich, contextualized knowledge that arises from the situation itself during the course of the clinical encounter.

It follows that the person best placed to conduct research into specific clinical nurse–patient encounters is the nurse (or, in certain cases, the patient). The most important and useful research methodologies for a science of the unique are therefore those that incorporate practitioner research in which nurses conduct on-the-spot inquiry into their own practice. Furthermore, the findings from practitioner research do not have to be written-up and published before they can be applied to practice but have the potential immediately to influence the clinical encounter from which they originated. A science of the unique is therefore an immediate and fully *reflexive* one that unites research and practice (and also researcher and practitioner) in the integrated act of *praxis* and results in wise action based on an intimate, rich, and contextual experiential knowledge of unique individual cases.

The rejection of technical rationality in favor of praxis does not merely *call into question* the relationship between the researcher and the practitioner; rather, it completely dissolves the distinction between them. Praxis is a form of on-the-spot experimentation that attempts to integrate research, theorizing, and practice into a single activity to be carried out by a practitioner-researcher in the clinical area. As such, it stands outside the mainstream of both the social science and the medical paradigms and draws on the traditions and epistemologies of more established practice disciplines such as education, psychotherapy, and political science. We can hear echoes in praxis of Karl Marx's dictum that "the philosophers have only interpreted the world, in various ways; the point is to change it" (Marx, 1845/1970, p. 123) and of Kurt Lewin's admonition that "research that produces nothing but books will not suffice" (Lewin, 1948, p. 203). The epistemology underpinning praxis is perhaps most succinctly summed up by Peter Reason under the rubric of "co-operative inquiry," which

> seeks knowledge in action for action. Co-operative researchers may write books and articles, but often the knowledge that is really important for them is the practical knowledge of new skills and abilities…. And thus in co-operative inquiry, education and social action may become fully integrated with the research process. (Reason, 1988, p. 13)

As Reason points out, the *process* involved in doing this type of research might include education and social action as well as data collection and therefore takes on a significance and importance far beyond what would be expected in traditional technical rational methodologies. In addition, the *outcome* is far wider in scope than mere books and articles, which, as Lewin tells us, simply will not do. The aims of praxis are *practical knowledge* and *practical change* for both the nurse *and* patient.

This is not intended to be a methods chapter, and, in any case, praxis is not defined by the data collection methods it employs, which can be many and varied (including quantitative methods) and which are chosen pragmatically to suit the task in hand. There are, however, a number of methodological approaches that are particularly suited to the aims of praxis, and these include participative and emancipatory action research, reflexive ethnography, single-case experiments, cooperative inquiry, and some approaches to reflective and reflexive practice. These methodologies share a number of features which make them particularly useful for nurses who wish to explore and improve their practice.

TOWARD SOME METHODOLOGICAL PRINCIPLES OF PRAXIS

1. Praxis, as we have seen, is a science of the unique and takes as its starting point the observation by the poet W. H. Auden (1967/1990) that "as persons, we are incomparable, unclassifiable, uncountable, irreplaceable" (p. 6). Thus, **praxis is a science of individual persons rather than a science of people as a collective whole**. I have argued above that while many of the qualitative social science methodologies purport to study individuals, most are concerned ultimately with generalizing or categorizing the findings to a wider population (statistical generalization) or to a general theory (analytic generalization). The methodologies

employed in praxis are concerned primarily with unique individual cases and no attempt is made to move from the specific to the general. We can see this approach, for example, in single-case experiments, which use mostly quantitative data collection methods to explore the effects of particular treatment or caring interventions on specific individual patients. Through careful pre- and post-testing, nurses are able to measure and modify the effects of their own interventions over time and thus to tailor individual care to meet the needs of their unique and individual patients. The purpose of single-case experiments is to learn about the unique needs and responses of individuals, and no attempt is made to generalize or transfer the findings between patients.

2. **Praxis places the practitioner-researcher at the heart of the research process.** Whereas many social and medical research methodologies could be described as practitioner-based, insofar as they include practitioners in the research process, perhaps collecting data or administering treatment interventions, praxis methodologies all involve the practitioner-researcher in the critical analysis of some aspect of the nurse's own practice. Praxis methodologies are therefore not merely practitioner-*based* but might be better described as practitioner-*centered*. The most fundamental and straightforward practitioner-centered research methodology is what Schön (1983) described as reflection-on-action, which entails a systematic and critical approach to thinking and writing about and learning from our own practice and, most importantly, applying what has been learned back into practice at the earliest opportunity.

3. We can see, then, that **praxis entails not only reflectivity but also reflexivity**, the application of research findings back into the practice setting from which they were gathered by the practitioner-researcher who gathered them. Reflexivity can be seen most clearly and overtly in Schön's (1983) other strategy for reflection, which he called reflection-*in*-action or on-the-spot experimenting. Reflection-in-action, in its most advanced form, involves a cyclical process of assessing the current situation, formulating a hypothesis, testing it through practical interventions and reevaluating the situation in the light of the intervention (Schön, 1983). This experimental cycle is conducted in the midst of practice by the practitioner-researcher as part of everyday *modus operandi*; it is, at the same time, a way of doing research and a way of doing nursing. As a cyclical process, reflection-in-action is both continuous (one cycle leads inexorably to the next) and continual (unlike most research methodologies, it has no termination point, for example, when the funding runs out). Reflection-in-action might therefore be regarded as the most fundamental and widely used methodology of praxis.

4. **The experimental approach described above is common to all of the methodologies employed in praxis.** For example, action research, as originally defined by Lewin (1948), "proceeds in a series of steps each of which is composed of a circle of planning, action, and fact-finding about the result of the action" (p. 206). In all cases, practitioner-researchers experiment with their practice by conducting a series of *systematic* and *controlled* treatment or caring interventions, which are then modified or revised according to what Lewin referred to above as "fact-finding about the result of the action."

5. While all practitioner-centered research is systematic and controlled, practitioner-researchers would generally reject the criterion of rigor that is much favored by social researchers. We have already seen that, in most social research methodologies, validity and reliability are guaranteed by rigorous adherence to method; in other words, the findings are to be trusted if and only if the prescribed method can be shown to have been followed rigorously and unswervingly. Practitioner research, however, is concerned less with valid and reliable findings than with positive action, and positive action depends on the reflexivity of the practitioner-researcher in responding to feedback as it arises. Whereas rigor implies rigidity and rule-following, **practitioner-researchers will value flexibility and rule bending (and, at times, rule breaking).** See, for example, Rolfe (2006b) for an account of research validity based on Lyotard's idea of rule-free judgments.

6. Finally, and perhaps most controversially, **practitioner-researchers reject the objective stance of the disinterested researcher.** They neither step back so as not to influence the "objects" of their research nor "bracket" their own preconceptions and leave them at the door. For example, cooperative inquirers actively engage with their "subjects" as partners in the research process and are thus fully immersed in the practice being studied. Stenhouse (1981) described the stance of the practitioner-researcher as "interested," not only in the sense of taking an interest in the issues and practices being researched but also in the sense of having a vested interest in the outcome of the research. Gadamer (1976) referred to this stance more straightforwardly as "prejudice" and regarded it not only as unavoidable but also as advantageous to the researcher. As Stenhouse argued, the first and foremost reason for conducting research into our own practice is to make things better, and we therefore have to exercise our professional judgment as to what constitutes improvement. For the practitioner-researcher, there is no objective, value-neutral viewpoint "out there" from which to conduct research. Like it or not, the nurse is fully immersed in the research-practice experience.

CONCLUSION

A number of writers have commented over the years on the existence of the so-called "theory–practice gap" in nursing. The blame for this gap between what theorists and researchers state *should* happen in practice and what *actually* happens is usually laid firmly at the feet of practitioners for not reading, understanding, and implementing the latest research findings. In this chapter, I have turned the tables by suggesting that the problem lies less with practice than with research, that the dominant nursing research methods and methodologies have not kept apace with changes in nursing practice, and that, subsequently, neither the methodologies themselves nor the findings derived from those methodologies are fit for the purpose of informing practicing nurses in the 21st century. I have further suggested that what is required is not simply a reconsideration and revision of the so-called "hierarchy of evidence" but rather a radical review of the technical rational relationship between research and practice.

The traditional technical rational paradigm of evidence-based practice regards research and clinical nursing as two separate and distinct activities, while generally failing to explicate in any detail just what links them, that is, what it might mean in practical terms for a nurse to *base* practice on the findings of large-scale statistical research. Rather than merely *basing* practice on research evidence, I have proposed a new epistemology of praxis that fully *integrates* the activities of research-gathering and nursing practice into a single, seamless activity undertaken by a single person, in which research and practice are constantly informing and responding to one another.

QUESTIONS FOR REFLECTION

1. Think about your own understanding of the term "evidence-based nursing." What do you consider to be the most useful and valuable sources of evidence for your own practice? What is it about these sources of evidence that makes them more useful to you?
2. Think of a recent case where you applied evidence in making a clinical, managerial, or other person-centered decision. Reflect on what was going through your mind as you weighed up the various pieces of evidence that contributed to your decision.
3. Think about some of the implications for practice and research of adopting a research paradigm based on a science of individual persons rather than collectively on people. How would the practices of nursing and research differ from the current paradigm? In particular, what would be the implications for patients of this new way of working?

REFERENCES

Anderson, E. R. (1973). *The role of the nurse*. London: Royal College of Nursing.

Auden, W. H. (1990). A short defense of poetry. In M. van Manen (Ed.), *Researching lived experience* (p. 6). New York: SUNY. (Original work published 1967)

Eliot, T. S. (1940). The rock. In T. S. Eliot (Ed.), *Collected poems* (pp. 107–127). London: Faber and Faber. (Original work published 1934)

Evidence-Based Medicine Working Group. (1992). Evidence-based medicine: A new approach to teaching the practice of medicine. *Journal of the American Medical Association, 268*, 2420–2425.

Fisher, R. A. (1935). *The design of experiments*. Edinburgh, UK: Oliver and Boyd.

French, B. (1998). Developing the skills required for evidence-based practice. *Nurse Education Today, 18*, 46–51.

Gadamer, H. G. (1976). *Philosophical hermeneutics*. Berkeley: University of California Press.

Giddens, A. (2009). *Sociology* (6th ed.). Cambridge, UK: Polity Press.

Greenwood, E. (1966). Attributes of a profession. In H. M. Vollmer & D. L. Mills (Eds.), *Professionalization* (pp. 10–19). Englewood Cliffs, NJ: Prentice-Hall.

Hammersley, M., & Atkinson, P. (1983). *Ethnography: Principles in practice.* London: Routledge.

International Council for Nurses. (2010). *Definition of nursing.* Retrieved December 1, 2010, from http://www.icn.ch/about-icn/icn-definition-of-nursing/

Kalisch, P. A., & Kalisch, B. J. (1995). *The advance of American nursing* (3rd ed.). Philadelphia: J.B. Lippincott.

Lewin, K. (1948). Action research and minority problems. In G. W. Lewin (Ed.), *Resolving social conflicts: Selected papers on group dynamics* (pp. 201–216). New York: Harper & Row.

Marx, K. (1970). Theses on Feuerbach. In K. Marx, F. Engels (Eds.), & C. J. Arthur (Trans.), *The German ideology* (pp. 121–123). London: Lawrence and Wishart. (Original work published 1845)

McLean, J. P. (1973). Nursing care study: Bilateral nephrectomy. *Nursing Mirror, 136*(10), 31–34.

Morton & Morton. (2003). *Evidence-based nursing practice.* Retrieved December 1, 2010, from http://www.ebnp.co.uk/The%20Hierarchy%20of%20Evidence.htm

Mulhall, A. (1998). Nursing, research and the evidence. *Evidence-Based Nursing, 1*(1), 4–6.

Nightingale, F. (1860). *Notes on nursing: What it is, and what it is not* (1st American ed.). New York: D. Appleton.

Polit, D. E., & Beck, C. T. (2004). *Nursing research: Principles and methods* (7th ed.). Philadelphia: Lippincott Williams & Wilkins.

Polit, D. E., & Beck, C. T. (2008). *Nursing research: Generating and assessing evidence for nursing practice* (8th ed.). Philadelphia: Lippincott Williams & Wilkins.

Polit, D. E., & Beck, B. P. (2006). *Essentials of nursing research: Methods, appraisal, and utilization* (6th ed.). Philadelphia: Lippincott Williams & Wilkins.

Priyjmachuk, S. (1996). A nursing perspective on the interrelationships between theory, research and practice. *Journal of Advanced Nursing, 23,* 679–684.

Royal College of Nursing. (1971). *Evidence to the Committee on Nursing.* London: Author.

Royal College of Nursing. (2010). *Defining nursing.* Retrieved December 1, 2010, from http://www.rcn.org.uk/__data/assets/pdf_file/0003/78564/001983.pdf

Reason, P. (1988). *Human inquiry in action.* London: Sage.

Rolfe, G. (2006a). Nursing praxis and the science of the unique. *Nursing Science Quarterly, 19*(1), 39–43.

Rolfe, G. (2006b). Judgments without rules: Towards a postmodern ironist concept of research validity. *Nursing Inquiry, 13,* 7–15.

Rolfe, G., & Gardner, L. (2005). Towards a nursing science of the unique: Evidence, reflexivity and the study of persons. *Journal of Research in Nursing, 10,* 297–310.

Sackett, D. L., Rosenberg, W. M. C., Gray, J. A. M., Haynes, R. B., & Richardson, W. S. (1996). Evidence based medicine: What it is and what it isn't. *British Journal of Medicine, 312,* 71–72.

Schön, D. (1983). *The reflective practitioner.* London: Temple Smith.

Stenhouse, L. (1978). Case study and case records: Towards a contemporary history of education. *British Educational Research Journal, 4*(2), 21–39.

Stenhouse, L. (1981). What counts as research? *British Journal of Educational Studies, 29*(2), 103–114.

INTERLUDE II

Mindfulness and Knowledge Development in Nursing Practice

Catherine Johnson
Pamela G. Reed

Nursing knowledge generation in the 21st century is radically changing from the research and theory development activities of the past. With the advent of the first universally acknowledged practice doctorate in nursing (the Doctor of Nursing Practice or DNP) and changing perspectives of evidence beyond that espoused by positivist philosophy, nursing practice experts are poised to become significant participants in knowledge development. We propose mindfulness as an approach that not only enhances patient care but also can open a space to expand awareness of oneself and the situation to facilitate knowledge development in the context of nursing practice. We invite you to explore the ideas presented here on mindfulness practice in reference to your own work in nursing.

Because of the constantly changing practice environment, research findings and extant theories can become outdated, perhaps quickly becoming no more than historical information about a point in time (Jarvis, 2000). Reflective practice is often described as a window through which previously unseen dynamics and implications for knowledge within the nurse–patient interaction can be revealed (Trelfa, 2005). However, mindfulness practice, not unlike the more familiar reflective practice, may enhance the knowledge we already obtain from extant research and theories to provide an evidence base that is more relevant to the changing practice context. Not until expert nurses unlock their own practice knowledge and theory generation process will full understanding of expert nursing practice be possible. Mindfulness practice can increase our understanding of clinical patterns and their meanings—as grounded in the expert nurse's beliefs and values, assessments and decisions, and knowledge and experiences.

MINDFULNESS AND EXPANDED AWARENESS

Over the past decade, mindfulness has garnered increased attention and supporting evidence across a variety of health-related disciplines (Christopher &

Maris, 2010). Jon Kabat-Zinn (1994), a pioneer of mindfulness practice, defined *mindfulness* as "paying attention in a particular way, on purpose, in the moment and non-judgmentally" (p. 4). Mindfulness practice also has been described as "open, undivided observation of what is occurring both internally and externally rather than a particular cognitive approach to external stimuli" (Brown & Ryan, 2003, p. 823). The mindful practitioner attends to his or her sensory and cognitive processes in a nonjudgmental way during everyday tasks to aid clarity and insight regarding their everyday reality. A strength of the mindful practitioner is an expanded capacity to maintain emotional balance within any particular life moment. To practice mindfulness is to cultivate awareness of being alive in the present moment (Solloway & Fisher, 2007). Deepening this awareness leads to being more present and experiencing life more vividly, yet also being aware of life's impermanent nature. Mindfulness, then, refers to an expanded awareness characterized by a purposeful and nonjudgmental attending to the present moment.

Paying attention is the prime objective of mindfulness. Through this process of discovery, you can observe your own experiences while participating in them. The correct attitude toward this process can be summarized by the words of Gunaratana (2002):

> *Never mind what I have been taught. Forget about theories and prejudgments and stereotypes...I want to understand the true nature of life. I want to know what this experience of being alive really is. I want to apprehend the true and deepest qualities of life, and I don't want to just accept somebody else's explanation. I want to see it for myself.* (p. 18)

All cultures in the world have a history of some mental practice designed to assist people in living and coping with the stresses of their world through increased understanding. These practices vary greatly but overall they include the elements of conscious thought, concentration, and reflection (Gunaratana, 2002). Within the Buddhist tradition, not only is concentration highly valued but equally so is the element of awareness that occurs with mindfulness.

INSIGHT MEDITATION

Vipassana, or insight meditation, is the oldest Buddhist meditation practice and involves the gradual cultivation of mindfulness or awareness. Some evidence suggests that Vipassana may be useful clinically although more research is indicated (Chiesa, 2010). With insight meditation, the meditator's attention is focused on certain aspects of her or his own experience through observation of the flow of life experiences moment to moment. Insight meditation is a mindfulness practice that focuses on breathing while sitting in a meditative state. There are mindfulness practices that involve other physical activities, which also aid in bringing mindfulness into everyday life. These include walking meditation or yoga postures. All are focused on developing awareness of "being in the body, with a mind" (Moss & Barnes, 2008, p. 12).

THE CHALLENGE OF CONCENTRATION

Insight meditation fosters development of mindfulness in part by increasing the ability for concentration. Concentration is regarded as a key tool in achieving enhanced awareness or mindfulness. Through this ancient form of sensitivity training, insight meditation helps a person become more receptive to life experiences by attentively listening, observing, and testing the reality experienced in the moment without judgment or bias. The enhanced concentration developed through meditation can become a natural approach to reflecting on your inner and external experiences in mindfulness practice.

The process of focusing on the realm of thoughts and the present moment is a daunting one. The mind is incredibly active, and if your focus is on paying attention to your senses, thoughts, and feelings in any given moment, you will soon be overwhelmed.

The concentration is not about being mindful of something in particular; to be mindful *of* something separates self from the present reality. Instead, the concentration has more to do with being mindful *in* the present. As Muho Noelke (2004) stated in a lecture he gave while he was the abbott at Antaiji, a Zen monastery:

> ... *We have to forget things like "I should be mindful of this or that." If you are mindful, you are already creating a separation...Don't be mindful, please! When you walk, just walk. Let the walk walk. Let the talk talk....Let the eating eat, the sitting sit, the work work. Let sleep sleep.*

For this reason, in the early stages of the meditative process, a focus on a concrete entity is especially helpful in maintaining concentration. As mentioned, a common entity used in insight meditation is the breath because breathing is a part of everyone's experience. This concentration on the breath in meditation is a tool to move you into the realm of the present moment and to achieve and sustain present-focused awareness or mindfulness.

RESEARCH ON MINDFULNESS

The Agency for Healthcare Research and Quality (AHRQ) published an evidence report in June 2007, *Meditation Practices for Health: State of Research*, indicating an increase in the prevalence of complementary mind–body therapeutic strategies that included mindfulness practice. Five categories of meditative practices were identified: mantra meditation, mindfulness meditation, yoga, Tai Chi, and Qi Gong. Mindfulness practices included mindfulness-based stress reduction (MBSR) and mindfulness-based cognitive therapy (MBCT), which researchers are studying for their therapeutic benefits to mental health. Universal to all types of meditative practices is concentration on awareness of breathing and control of attention.

Results from the AHRQ (2007) analysis failed to demonstrate positive benefits on clinical outcomes of patients with hypertension, cardiovascular disease, or substance abuse. However, within healthy populations, meditative practices, including mindfulness meditation, had positive health benefits. The strongest and most consistent physiological effect of meditative practices was reduction of heart rate, blood pressure, and cholesterol. The strongest neurophysiological effect identified was an increase in verbal creativity. Overall, the effectiveness of mindfulness on stress reduction, well-being, and other psychological and physiological states has been well documented (e.g., Greeson, 2008).

Research by Solloway and Fisher (2007) into the measurement and effects of mindfulness practice generated results that may have implications for developing nursing knowledge in practice. Their study involved 338 undergraduate students and a comparison over time and across two groups, those who received mindfulness training and those who did not receive the training. Methodological results indicated that mindfulness is "teachable, learnable and amenable to measurement" (Solloway & Fisher, p. 69). Substantive findings suggested that mindfulness training in novice practitioners effects an increase in "psychological strengths," including increased emotional balance, being a more attentive listener, feeling more positive about accomplished tasks, noticing things in nature never noticed previously, increased insight, and increased ability to examine life without being caught up in the process (Solloway & Fisher, 2007, pp. 70–71). These effects of mindfulness practice are of interest because they may facilitate nurses' abilities to see new concepts and make connections that might otherwise be missed in the clinical situation. The positive impact of meditation and mindfulness on learning and perceiving may have implications in helping nurses become cognizant of their personal theories and develop concepts relevant to their clinical practice.

OUTCOMES OF MINDFULNESS IN NURSING PRACICE

In mindfulness practice, one becomes aware of the present moment and every thought and feeling as an inner monologue emerges. Mindfulness practice creates an attentive, intelligent quality in each element of one's experience, yet does not focus on "figuring it out"; rather, the mindful nurse merely observes these parts of experience in a nonjudgmental way. The capacity of simply being aware and accepting the present moment is the desired outcome of mindfulness practice. Openness to the flow of thought and increased attention to the present moment occur as one practices mindfulness. Unexpected outcomes, fears, or desires are acknowledged but are not dwelled upon as one increases appreciation of the quiet wisdom within.

An important outcome of mindfulness is the development of compassion, a critical element of caring. Mindfulness has been described as a purification of the mind, particularly in reference to ego processes of greed and hatred. Transformational exercises are often used to prepare the meditator with a mantra of "universal loving kindness" (Gunaratana, 2002). This exercise includes speaking the following intention prior to meditation practice and repeating it in full, focusing on your self and then on your teachers, relatives, friends, enemies, and last on all living beings:

May I live well, happy and peaceful. May no harm come to me. May no difficulties come to me. May no problems come to me. May I always meet with success.

May my teachers live well, happy and peaceful. May no harm come to them. May no difficulties come to them. May no problems come to them. May they always meet with success. . . . [and so on in reference to others.]. (Gunaratana, 2002, p. 4)

These Universal Loving Kindness Intentions are meant to guide you as the meditator in transformation of your speech and actions toward yourself and all living beings and to prepare you for meditation and mindfulness practice.

Insight meditation facilitates development of mindfulness. However, mindfulness is not contained in the meditative process only. Mindfulness can be cultivated in the context of everyday life through gentle reminders to maintain awareness of whatever is happening moment to moment. Mindfulness provides a clearer perspective of both your self and your situation.

There are both personal and professional benefits to be gained by engaging in this meditative process. Within your personal life, you may experience increased calm and satisfaction in the world around you when you focus on the quiet contemplation of meditation and on the Universal Loving Kindness Intentions. In the professional realm, you may find yourself more available to your patients, interacting with them in a calm, compassionate manner.

POTENTIAL KNOWLEDGE-BASED OUTCOMES

Mindfulness practice is a strategy to enrich nursing practice and increase opportunities for nurses to develop theoretical ideas out of their professional practice. Mindfulness can facilitate knowledge development in nursing practice through awareness and integration of various ways of knowing in nursing, such as that involved in the personal theories Rolfe (1998) suggested are developed by expert nurses in practice.

Developing personal theory in practice must involve personal knowledge—that is, awareness of your philosophy of nursing and beliefs about practice—and all nurses possess a philosophy whether or not they have articulated it. Trelfa (2005) advised that reflective practice cannot be divorced from the professional's beliefs and feelings but is linked to one's worldview and practice philosophy. Avis and Freshwater (2006) urge careful examination of practitioners' beliefs and thought processes, all viewed as influences in their interpretation of evidence and the resultant decisions made in practice. In addition, the Buddhist practice of insight meditation as it supports mindfulness practice can help nurses to break down these complex thought processes through expanded awareness of their sensory and cognitive experiences.

New mental habits can be attained through the ongoing practice of meditation and subsequent ability to deal with conscious thought and sensory experiences. When practicing mindful, nonjudgmental awareness of your surroundings and nursing actions, you as the nurse may see areas for enhancing your own professional development as well as for improving the effectiveness of patients' own health care strategies. Professional health care providers, then, are challenged to use mindfulness practice to explore and articulate emotional and cognitive elements of their practice and then revisit these definitions in light of new self-awareness. The following scenario is an example of how mindfulness practice helped Dr. Johnson gain awareness of the emotional and theoretical elements embedded in a challenging clinical situation.

EXAMPLE OF MINDFULNESS PRACTICE IN A CONTEXT OF VIOLENCE

For the practicing nurse, the process of mindfulness may parallel processes you already have experienced. Expert nurses often may see beyond the nursing theories they have been taught to perceive their clinical situations *in the moment* as a natural flow of the elements they seek to understand. In what is often described as an intuitive process, they see the *whole* and react to the situation in a comprehensive way. This perception is very similar to mindfulness in that expert nurses break away from the previously described experiences of others and trust their own perceptions and insights. In doing this, they identify and link together pertinent concepts, building their own theories to explain what is occurring in the present moment. Practicing nurses' personal theories evolve out of heightened awareness of this moment and the simultaneous integration of knowledge about the underlying process taking place.

I (CJ) experienced this awareness in my practice as a family nurse practitioner in Deming, New Mexico. I had been practicing mindfulness meditation for some time and was becoming increasingly aware of moment-to-moment experiences that I felt as energy flowing around me. Several incidents of violence had occurred both in our clinic and in the small community of Deming. I, along with the clinic staff, felt anxious and unsafe.

As I became increasingly mindful through daily meditation, I began to feel less anxiety and more comfortable and at peace. I also experienced an increase in my nonjudgmental awareness of the situation, which resulted in an increase in my effectiveness as a team member and practitioner. My acceptance of the situation and my awareness of my own anxiety and that of the other staff members helped me talk more freely with my teammates about these feelings and how they might have an impact on our patients. We as a team were then able to look at our clients as part of the same environment we were experiencing and its influence on all of us. As I became more a part of the present experienced by my clients, I could purposefully include this shared awareness in my assessments, decisions, and plans. I increased my ability to provide compassionate care by being in the present moment with myself, my teammates, and my clients. Together, we joined in the present and became more at peace, supported, and effective.

My mindfulness practice involved a reflecting-*in*-practice that increased my awareness and understanding of the situation and enhanced my actions with clients and my team. Next, as a second step in using mindfulness to develop nursing knowledge, I reflected on this scenario, a kind of reflection-*on*-practice, to further explicate and refine what began as my personal theory that emerged in the situation. Here is my stream of theoretical ideas from my personal theory:

- Mindfulness practice helped me reflect on a problematic situation and gain increased awareness of my own anxiety.
- Increased awareness facilitated my open discussion of concerns among the team.
- This open discussion, in turn, helped the team and me perceive clients as part of the same environment and as having similar anxieties and fears.
- This perception enabled me to purposefully share my perceptions with clients and obtain a fuller assessment of their concerns in the process.
- This perception also enhanced my compassion toward clients and my ability to convey this to clients.
- Expanded knowledge of the situation coupled with my compassionate approach in my nursing practice led to more effective interventions and better teamwork in the clinic.

NEXT STEPS

A next step in building nursing knowledge is to connect existing theory and research and other practitioners' experiences with my personal theory. I would use these sources to support or challenge the string of inferences I drew from my clinical observations and reflections, and to identify key concepts that may be linked together to organize a theoretical framework. The framework would propose an explanation of what was happening in that clinical situation. This framework would be generated from a synthesis of all the available evidence. It would then be tested through research methods and by practicing nurses who share a similar concern with enhancing health care provider well-being, teamwork, and client care in the context of threats of violence.

Thus, through the practice of mindfulness, nurses can achieve greater understanding of their environment and their practice, specifically through the tools of concentration and heightened awareness of self and the clinical situation. Mindfulness practice not only increases the number of elements that nurses factor into their clinical strategies and actions but also widens the opportunities for identifying new concepts that may better explain clinical phenomena. Mindfulness practice enables the nurse to take a crucial mental step away from the clinical situation to perceive all of the elements involved in a situation and in the actions taken and to evaluate clinical dynamics and outcomes. This understanding not only contributes to our practice wisdom but also provides opportunity for concept and theory development.

A STEP-BY-STEP GUIDE FOR INSIGHT MEDITATION
LEADING TO MINDFULNESS

The following is a step-by-step guide to participating in insight meditation (Gunaratana, 2002). Meditation is an experience that is learned through experience and practice. Guidance through this process by a knowledgeable teacher is required for greatest success.

1. Dress in loose soft clothing that will not restrict circulation. No belts or thick material. Shoes and socks or stockings should be taken off.
2. Traditional Asian postures are sitting on the floor with a cushion to elevate the spine. A chair can be used, however. Focus of posture is to choose one that allows you to remain immobile without pain for the entire length of the meditation.
3. Determine how long you are going to meditate based on how long you can sit immobile without pain. Beginners should begin with not more than 20 minutes of meditation. Time is not the focus for success; progress is.
4. After positioning yourself and sitting motionless, close your eyes.
5. Share your Universal Loving Kindness Intentions
6. Take three deep breaths, then breathe normally, letting your breath flow in and out freely. Focus your attention on the *rim of your nostrils*. Simply notice the *feeling of breath* going in and out. These are the **first two objects** of focus for meditation.
7. Ignore any thought, memory, sound, smell, or taste. Focus exclusively on the breath.
8. As you continue, you will notice that initially the inhalation and exhalation is short and rapid but with increased awareness you will notice it becoming longer as your mind and body become calm.
9. As you continue, you will begin to notice that the entire breathing process becomes more subtle. A calm and peaceful feeling of breathing will come.
10. Despite your best efforts, your mind may wander and you may be focused on your friends, your family, bills you need to pay, and so on. As soon as you notice you are no longer focused on your breath, return to a focus on the rim of your nostrils and your inhalation and exhalation. Counting can be used to assist you in staying focused. For example, you can count 1–1–1–1 with the next inhalation and 2–2–2–2 with the next exhalation. Continue up to 5 cycles counting up to 10. Repeat as needed until your breathing is quiet and barely noticed.
11. As the breath gets more quiet and subtle, your mind and body can feel so light it feels like you are floating. You will begin to be aware of an *image or sensation* which is a sign of meditation and is the **third object** of meditation. This may appear as a star, the moon, a long string, or film of clouds. It is unique to you and it means you have reached the state of concentration sufficient for insight meditation and mindfulness.
12. At the end of the meditation session (indicated by the sound of a bell in some settings), you will slowly open your eyes and be aware of the environment. You will feel calm and peaceful. Move carefully and quietly as this is a transition period that must be taken slowly.

With consistent and patient practice, you can develop deepening levels of concentration that will increase your ability to develop mindfulness. This building process may take months to years, and for most meditators, it is a lifelong quest.

However, soon after initiating the mediation practice, you can experience results by an increase in peacefulness and calm (Gunaratana, 2002).

MINDFULNESS AND THE FUTURE OF SCHOLARLY PRACTICE

We have proposed mindfulness as a strategy to enrich nursing practice and increase opportunities for nurses to develop theoretical ideas out of their professional practice. Similarly, Sigma Theta Tau International (Freshwater, Horton-Deutsch, Sherwood, & Taylor, 2005) promotes meditation and mindfulness practice as a strategy to promote reflective practice, proposed as an overall means to "encourage deeper levels of analysis and interpretation of nursing issues relating to practice ..." (p. 3). The practice of insight meditation and the development of expanded concentration through mindfulness practice enable nurses to examine their thoughts, decisions, knowledge base, and feelings and reflect on the entire process within a patient–nurse interaction. Mindfulness, as a process similar to Schön's (1983) reflection-in-action, can increase nurses' capacities to attend to patients' needs and enhance practice knowledge in their constantly changing practice environments (Freshwater et al., 2005). From this new level of awareness *in* practice as well as from later reflections *on* practice, nurses can evaluate and refine their own knowledge base and improve clinical practice.

Research is needed to better understand the potential for mindfulness to promote scholarly practice, specifically the impact of mindfulness on the nurse's awareness and use of personal theories to extend concept and theory development in nursing. Mindfulness has the potential to provide both the individual nurse and the profession a means to better understand the complex practice environment of nursing care and the reality of nursing practice within this environment. Exploration of mindfulness as a knowledge-enhancing process may provide critical insights into the practice wisdom of expert nurses, as nursing expands its practice boundaries with the practice doctorate and seeks to identify and measure the unique contributions of this new role in nursing.

QUESTIONS FOR REFLECTION

1. Reflecting on the mindfulness practice example, what theoretical ideas might you identify?
2. What nursing experiences have you had in which mindfulness practice might be useful in promoting your own or clients' well-being?
3. The chapter outlined a guide for insight meditation leading to mindfulness practice that can be followed by DNP and PhD nurses. How might you use insight meditation in your own practice to move nursing knowledge forward in a new way?
4. What are some of the challenges you might face when engaging in mindfulness practice to provide patient care and build knowledge?

REFERENCES

Agency for Healthcare Research and Quality. (2007). *Meditation practices for health: State of the research* (AHRQ Publication No. 07-E010). Washington, DC: U.S. Government Printing Office.

Avis, M., & Freshwater, D. (2006). Evidence for practice, epistemology and critical reflection. *Nursing Philosophy, 7*, 216–224.

Brown, K. W., & Ryan, R. M. (2003). The benefits of being present: Mindfulness and its role in psychological well-being. *Journal of Personality and Social Psychology, 84*, 822–848.

Chiesa, A. (2010). Vipassana meditation: Systematic review of current evidence. *Journal of Alternative and Complementary Medicine, 16*(1), 37–46.

Christopher, J. C., & Maris, J. A. (2010). Integrating mindfulness as self-care into counseling and psychotherapy training. *Counseling and Psychotherapy Research, 10*(2), 114–125.

Freshwater, D., Horton-Deutsch, S., Sherwood, G., & Taylor, B. (2005). *Position paper on the scholarship of reflective practice.* Indianapolis, IN: Sigma Theta Tau International. Retrieved from http://www.nursingsociety.org/aboutus/PositionPapers/Documents/resource_reflective.doc

Greeson, J. M. (2008). Mindfulness research update: 2008. *Complementary Health Practice Review, 14*(1), 10–18.

Gunaratana, H. (2002). *Mindfulness in plain English.* Somerville, MA: Wisdom.

Jarvis, P. (2000). The practitioner-researcher in nursing. *Nurse Education Today, 20*, 30–35.

Kabat-Zinn, J. (1994). *Wherever you go there you are: Mindful meditation in everyday life.* New York: Hyperion.

Moss, D., & Barnes, R. (2008). Birdsong and footprints: Tangibility and intangibility in a mindfulness research project. *Reflective Practice, 9*(1), 11–12.

Noelke, M. (2004, October). Adult practice 18: Stop being mindful. *Lotus in the fire.* Shin'onsen, Japan: Antaiji. Retrieved from http://antaiji.dogen-zen.de/eng/adult18.shtml

Rolfe, G. (1998). *Expanding nursing knowledge: Understanding and researching your own practice.* Oxford, UK: Butterworth Heinemann.

Schön, D. A. (1983). *The reflective practitioner: How professionals think in action.* New York: Basic Books.

Solloway, S., & Fisher, W. (2007). Mindfulness in measurement: Reconsidering the measureable in mindfulness practice. *International Journal of Transpersonal Studies, 26*, 58–81.

Trelfa, J. (2005). Faith in reflective practice. *Reflective Practice, 6*, 205–212.

Creating a Nursing Intervention out of a Passion for Theory and Practice

Nelma B. Crawford Shearer

*T*here is considerable literature on how to develop nursing interventions. Some instruct that nursing interventions are developed from a systematic review of literature to link the identified problem or phenomena of concern with research efforts (Polit & Hungler, 1995). Others emphasize that theory drives the development of an intervention (e.g., Sidani & Braden, 1998; Whittemore & Grey, 2002). My focus here, however, is to discuss an extension of typical approaches used in the development of theory-based interventions, to show you an approach that emphasizes practice. It is an iterative or developmental process in which practice enriches theory and serves as a guide in creating theory-based interventions. This chapter chronicles my work in developing a theory-based nursing intervention on health empowerment as an example of how nurses may develop their own ideas into theory-based interventions. My doctoral studies were the catalyst for heightening my awareness of the link between practice and theory. The process began in doctoral school, by considering all that I was learning along with my practice experiences.

Developing a theory-based intervention is not a linear process. It is a back-and-forth, iterative process that reflects on practice experiences and considers theoretical ideas and research findings. A metatheory course enabled me to examine the nature and function of theory and strategies to build it, which set the foundation for what would become a theory-based intervention. Theory came alive as I reflected on practice experiences and linked ideas with my philosophy of nursing and other factors that play a role in how I view the world. A course in middle-range theory captured the importance of merging personal practice experiences with mental pictures to better understand a special or particular theoretical concept of my own creation, as it related to other established nursing concepts. This course also helped me better understand critical links between theory, practice, and research. From these foundational courses, I developed and tested the health empowerment theory through qualitative and quantitative work. The process culminated in what I call the intervention stage of my theory development, when I tested the theory-based intervention with homebound older women.

REFLECTING ON PRACTICE EXPERIENCES

Nursing practice provides a foundation for knowledge production (Reed, 2006). These practice experiences may lay dormant, however, until the nurse learns about the process of inquiry. This happened for me during my 1st year of doctoral education, which reawakened past clinical experiences that provided data for my theory building.

Practice Example 1: During my undergraduate clinical practice experience in community health, I visited a woman on her family farm. The woman had been in a car accident and suffered a fracture to her hip. She was able to move around her home with the use of crutches but was not able to stand on her feet for a long time. While completing the assessment, it became apparent that what was bothering her most was the need to organize her kitchen to prepare family meals. This meant rearranging her kitchen cupboards and moving items to within-chair-level reach. I stopped and asked myself: *Should I rearrange her kitchen to make it more manageable; would this be perceived as a nursing role?* I did rearrange the woman's kitchen, and in retrospect, I enacted a tacit nursing theory about health that helped this woman live according to what was meaningful and healthy to her in the context of her health concerns. For this woman, health was defined as being able to prepare meals for her family, and for me, nursing was defined as facilitating her ability to purposefully participate in attaining this meaningful goal. This encounter links to my current theory of practice, the enactment of which empowers individuals to purposefully participate in change and in so doing provides knowledge for nurses to directly intervene in the situation.

Practice Example 2: After graduation, I worked in a rural hospital to polish my technical skills. One afternoon, I began making rounds and encountered an older female patient who was crying. As I tried to comfort her, she told me a story about her daughter and how she had drowned in a flash flood. Despite the fact that I should have been passing afternoon medications to a variety of patients, I took the time to sit with her, listen to her story, and stayed with her until she stopped crying. When I got ready to leave, she graciously thanked me for listening and told me that sharing her daughter's story made her feel better. She commented that she knew I had more important things to do for other patients. Reflecting on this experience later during my doctoral studies, I realized that listening and providing support as well as helping individuals find ways to help themselves were components of my emerging theory of health empowerment.

Practice Example 3: Through my teaching experiences in a large metropolitan clinic, I often witnessed nurses creating a standardized plan of care for the sick children rather than working with the mother to create a personalized care plan specific to her children. The mothers were not always able to follow through with the standardized plan of care and returned to the clinic because the children's health had not improved. Nurses often grumbled about the returning mothers' failure to follow the plan of care and labeled them *frequent fliers* and noncompliant. In fact, the nurses appeared puzzled when the mothers consistently failed to adhere to the prescribed plan of care for their children. Reflecting back and guided by my theory of practice, the mothers should not have been prescribed standardized care plans. Instead, their children should have been given individualized plans based on nurse and mother working together and on the child's needs.

CLARIFYING MY PHILOSOPHIC WORLDVIEW

An initial formal step in my theory work occurred—unbeknown to me at the time— that involved articulating my philosophy of nursing science. Through coursework, exploration of my values and beliefs, and reflection on practice experiences, I formalized my personal philosophy of nursing. In particular, readings and discussions about the contextual-dialectic worldview from Pepper (1948) and the lifespan developmental literature (Lerner, 1997) and Parse's (1987) simultaneity and Newman's (1992) unitary-transformative worldviews from nursing helped clarify my philosophic views. The *contextual-dialectic worldview* focuses on the dynamic relationship between person and the environment; people are active in concert with an active environment and are capable of growing in the midst of conflict. *Lifespan development* is an ongoing historical event that has the potential for qualitative as well as quantitative change. The *simultaneity paradigm* presents human beings as synergistic with the environment, and health is individually defined. The *unitary-transformative worldview* focuses on human beings as integral with their environment, identified by pattern and not biopsychosocial parts, and changing in ways that are not deterministic, that is, that cannot be controlled or predicted with much accuracy.

CONCEPT ANALYSIS AND CLARIFICATION

The concept *empowerment* captured my interest during my earlier practice experiences. I witnessed women who experienced frustration after being prescribed standardized care rather than receiving a personalized care plan. From my philosophical perspective, the women should have been listened to, supported, and encouraged to actively participate in developing their treatment plan. To better understand the concept of empowerment by focusing on health rather than illness, I searched the literature in nursing, health promotion, psychology, and social work. The selection of literature was also influenced by my nursing worldview, values, beliefs, and assumptions. As a contextual thinker, I recognized that my perceptions and observations were influenced by the setting, particularly by my interactions with the patient and environment.

The concept analysis and clarification involved two phases, both of which, it is important to note, were influenced by my worldview. The first phase followed Walker and Avant's (2005) guidelines in which attributes, antecedents, and outcomes are identified from a synthesis of the research and theory literature. As one result of this phase, I identified attributes of empowerment as belief in self, personal strengths and abilities, choice, control over factors affecting one's life, recognition, transformation, resources, and a desire or willingness to take action as participation in change.

In the second phase, I formulated statements of association and conditional relationships between my concept and other concepts to assist me in forming the skeleton of my emerging theory of health empowerment (Walker & Avant, 2005). In statements of associational relationship, I proposed that empowerment was positively associated with personal control, high self-esteem, autonomy, health and well-being as well as levels of control over life, consciousness, participation, and relationship. Conditional statements identified empowerment as linked to people and resources and a sense of personal competence with willingness to take action. Also, in reviewing the literature on empowerment, I found that the term was generally associated with increased self-esteem, self-worth, inner confidence, and well-being and was viewed as a process involving relationships. Two very different assumptions surfaced during the review. Some authors viewed empowerment as an inherent developmental process, whereby empowerment included levels or steps, and a person became increasingly empowered. Others viewed empowerment as a social process in which empowerment occurred as a result of external forces acting on the individual and affecting the individual's sense of control and feeling of power (Shearer & Reed, 2004).

DEFINITION OF EMPOWERMENT

As a result of the initial analysis and statement clarification, I defined empowerment as *the extent to which one's developmental process, beginning with a conscious choice in the face of a meaningful health event, facilitates a transforming belief in self*. Empowerment is viewed as an inherent process in which the woman "inpowers" self.

RESEARCH

QUALITATIVE WORK

Building on the findings of the concept analysis, I conducted qualitative research using *phenomenological methods* to discover the meaning of the lived experience of feeling in control of health among women with children. I focused on women because I viewed women as gatekeepers of their family health and believed that women who viewed themselves as in control could better care for themselves as well as their family.

From the findings, I identified processual variables of empowerment. That is, health empowerment in women began with a memorable health event. Then, throughout the experience, self-talk served to encourage the woman to take action for health and life. Both self-talk and social support served to reinforce proof that

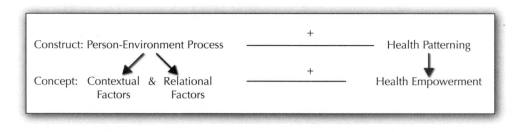

FIGURE 6.1
Conceptual Model.

she was in control and had a choice. There were instances when social support from significant others was required, as though to boost her sense of empowerment. The supportive relationship provided the "electrical current"—the charge needed to remain in control.

To guide me in the development of a theoretical model, I drew a picture linking the relationships that emerged from my qualitative work and coursework, along with my practice experiences. Based on the findings, I created a conceptual model that depicted a person–environment process as positively associated with health patterning and the two broad concepts, *contextual factors* and *interpersonal factors*, as positively associated with health empowerment as an outcome (Figure 6.1).

QUANTITATIVE WORK

Findings of the qualitative study provided foundational work to *develop and test a theoretical framework or model of health empowerment in women using a descriptive correlation design* (Shearer, 2004). My framework was influenced broadly by my worldview, adult developmental theory, and Rogers' (1992) science of unitary human beings, particularly the principle of integrality depicting human beings as integral with their environment in their daily living and health experience. For women, health empowerment was viewed as a developmental task in that person–environment interactions are central to developmental progress and well-being (Lerner, 1997; Reed, 1983). Accordingly, Rogers' principle of integrality suggests that health empowerment involves both person and environmental factors. The woman is seen as a person in mutual process with the nurse viewed as representing a significant element in her environment. I theorized that a partnership between the nurse and woman evolves from a health-seeking event.

To test my health empowerment framework (Shearer, 2004), I proposed positive relationships between the *person–environment* (evolving, ever changing unitary [or mutual] process of human beings and environment) and *health-patterning* (dynamic process of assisting patients to purposefully participate in change). Person–environment and health-patterning were the two broad constructs in my theory. Under each construct, I identified less abstract concepts that could be measured in testing the theory. *Person–environment* was conceptualized in terms of two concepts: (a) **contextual factors** (operationalized by personal profile characteristics including age, income, years of education, number of children, and years married) and (b) **relational factors** (operationalized as social support and professional support) that reflect Rogers' (1992) integrality in terms of mutual interaction, support, and mutual change of the woman and others. *Health patterning* was conceptualized in terms of one concept: health empowerment (operationalized as sense of power as a *knowing participation in change* [Barrett & Caroselli, 1998) and as health promoting lifestyle behaviors [Pender, 1996]).

I tested my framework in a sample of 123 women, aged 21 to 45. Results suggested 43% of the variance in health empowerment (indexed as health promoting lifestyle behaviors) was explained by level of education and the relational factor, social support. In addition, 38% of the variance in health empowerment (indexed as sense of power as a *knowing participation in change*) was explained by social support (Shearer, 2004). Study findings partially supported the theoretical framework consistent with assumptions that empowerment emerges from the person–environment mutual process. The limited explanatory ability of contextual and relational factors, however, highlighted the need to explore this area further.

At this juncture in my research and practice career, I became involved with the older adult population through my community health practice and experiences with my own aging parents (Shearer, 2002). Personal experiences as well as professional practice influenced perspectives guiding my research and thinking. I recognized that I needed to return to qualitative research to better understand the contextual and relational factors explaining empowerment. My population of interest was community-dwelling older women.

QUALITATIVE WORK

In a study using focus groups with community-dwelling older women, I further refined my understanding of social supportive needs and resources facilitating health empowerment (Shearer & Fleury, 2006). Focus group data provided a detailed description of the social and contextual factors used to facilitate health empowerment. I clarified that *social supportive resources* fostered health empowerment by providing encouragement as well as information and feedback in negotiating life changes within the aging process. The contextual factors that I previously viewed as personal characteristics were now viewed as *contextual resources* characterized by community and organizational structures providing social service resources to the participants at a system level. Based on this qualitative study, I refined the concept of *environment* within the health empowerment framework to reflect social-contextual resources. Social-contextual resources connoted perceived supportive relationships and opportunities for nurturance and the exchange of information and material to foster health empowerment.

In a final qualitative study, I used phenomenological methodology to discover the lived experience of health empowerment in homebound older women and to clarify dimensions of personal resources and social and contextual resources facilitating empowerment in this population (Shearer, 2007). Qualitative data highlighted social-contextual resources and, more importantly, the importance of personal

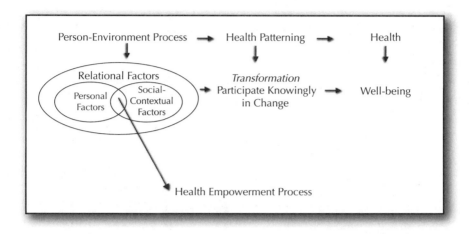

FIGURE 6.2

Theoretical Framework.

resources. *Personal resources* reflected the unique characteristics of the woman, such as inherent strength as self-capacity that promoted change and growth. *Social-contextual resources* such as social contacts and supportive networks identified by the participants enhanced the women's ability to stay connected and remain in their own homes, thus providing the basis for proposing my intervention.

I used the findings from the qualitative studies to revise and refine the health empowerment theoretical framework to include *personal resources* (initially called contextual factors) and *social-contextual resources* (initially called relational factors). I arrived at a view of health empowerment as a relational process emerging from the woman's *recognition* of personal resources and social-contextual resources (Shearer, 2007). Through the health empowerment process, a transformation occurred in the woman's awareness of and belief in her ability to knowingly participate in the changes inherent of health and health outcomes. This view involved a shift from a paternalistic perspective in which the health care provider establishes the goals to one where the homebound older woman purposefully participates in determining and progressing toward attainment of personal health goals, thus promoting well-being (Figure 6.2).

QUANTITATIVE WORK—INTERVENTION STUDY

I conceived the *health empowerment intervention* (HEI), guided by my theory of health empowerment (Shearer, 2000, 2004, 2009), as a way to develop and expand clinical knowledge. From my practice and research experiences, I found that women, particularly homebound older women, were at risk for losing their independence as their health needs became more complex and their ability to achieve their health goals seemed to be limited because they were unaware of resources. To enhance a homebound woman's health empowerment, I proposed that she first had to become aware of her resources, specifically *personal resources* and *social-*

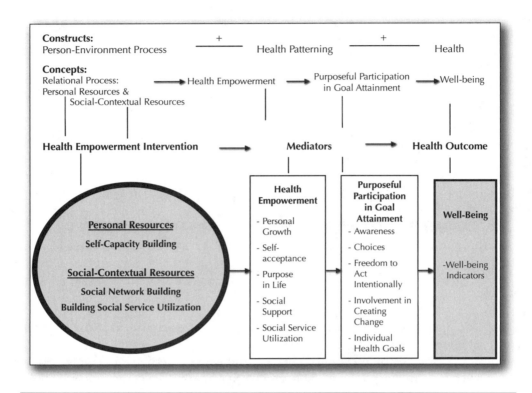

FIGURE 6.3

Health Empowerment Intervention Framework.

contextual resources. Figure 6.3 depicts the HEI framework, the variables and their relationships within the health empowerment theoretical framework and the intervention mechanisms (Shearer, Fleury, & Belyea, 2010).

TRANSLATING THE HEI TO PRACTICE

From a practice perspective, the focus of the HEI was to address the homebound older woman's personally relevant health goals and means to attain these goals. The nurse in concert with the woman facilitates the engagement of the woman in the process of recognizing personal resources, including self-capacity, and social contextual resources, including social network and access to social services. In addition, the HEI addressed personally relevant health goals and concerns for each homebound older woman and the means to attain these goals (Shearer, 2009).

Practice encounters that are guided by the theory of health empowerment and the HEI involve facilitating health on the women's terms and in the context of the moment (Shearer, Fleury, & Reed, 2009). A nurse practicing from a health empowerment perspective promotes the woman's awareness of and engagement in personal and social contextual resources first and foremost by listening to her (Practice

Example 2). Nursing actions are then directed at helping an older woman become aware of and use resources to purposefully participate in working toward the attainment of health goals (Practice Examples 1, 2, and 3). Thus, the nurse in concert with the older woman engages in a participatory process in which the nurse listens and encourages the older adult to talk, share, and enact her health goals (Shearer, 2009).

In actual practice, the nurse would focus on helping the woman recall and/or build awareness of *personal resources* through constructive reminiscence of a time when the woman felt able to overcome a challenge. Reminiscence can be thought of as memory release in which life experiences are poured out and used to facilitate self-capacity building through the acknowledgement of strengths. One strategy a nurse would use to increase awareness of *social-contextual resources* is facilitating problem-solving methods to help the woman identify persons and community resources that supported her in the past. Building on this recognition, the woman then accesses and engages new resources to attain her health care goals. In addition, role-playing facilitates reconnecting with others, seeking needed help, and contacting and communicating with social service agencies to access needed resources (Shearer, 2009).

THE INTEGRALITY OF MY RESEARCH, PRACTICE, AND THEORY-BASED INTERVENTION

The theory-based HEI unfolded as a developmental process whereby practice enriched my theorizing and served as a guide in creating the intervention. Explicating my theory-based intervention did not occur overnight nor was it guided by a single design or research method. I used multiple and diverse research methods to develop the intervention. It was important to clarify my philosophic views and beliefs in developing my theory, given my passion for promoting well-being in vulnerable populations and for understanding—from a nursing perspective—the human health experience.

In my ongoing program of research, I will continue to focus on an understanding of person and environmental factors that facilitate health empowerment, resulting in health outcomes. Given my dual passions for practice and theory, it is gratifying that my research goals lead to new ways of linking practice with theory and to discovering how theory can enrich practice. New thinking in this direction will help promote an awareness of the full spectrum of factors that may optimize health of older adults.

QUESTIONS FOR REFLECTION

1. What practice experiences have left their footprints in your mind?
2. What are you passionate about in nursing, is it theory, practice, research, or a combination?
3. How do you see yourself becoming a scholar and creator of a theory-based intervention?

REFERENCES

Barrett, E., & Caroselli, C. (1998). Methodological ponderings related to the power as knowing participation in change tool. *Nursing Science Quarterly*, 11, 17–21.

Lerner, R. (1997). *Concepts and theories of human development* (2nd ed.). Mahway, NJ: Lawrence Erlbaum.

Newman, M. A. (1992). Prevailing paradigms in nursing. *Nursing Outlook, 40*, 10–13, 32.

Parse, R. (1987). Paradigms and theories. In R. Parse (Ed.), *Nursing science: Major paradigms, theories, and critiques* (pp. 1–11). Philadelphia: Saunders.

Pender, N. (1996). *Health promotion in nursing practice* (3rd ed.). Stamford, CT: Appleton & Lange.

Pepper, S. P. (1948). *World hypotheses: A study in evidence.* Berkeley: University of California Press.

Polit, D. F., & Hungler, B. P. (1995). *Nursing research: Principles and methods* (5th ed.). Philadelphia: Lippincott.

Reed, P. (1983). Implications of the life-span developmental framework for well-being in adulthood and aging. *Advances in Nursing Science, 6*, 18–25.

Reed, P. G. (2006). The practice turn in nursing epistemology. *Nursing Science Quarterly, 19*(1), 51–60.

Rogers, M. E. (1992). Nursing science and space age. *Nursing Science Quarterly, 5*, 27–34.

Shearer, N. B. C. (2000). Facilitators of health empowerment in women (AAT 9965911; Doctoral dissertation, University of Arizona, 2000). *Dissertation Abstracts International, 861*(03), pp. 1–144.

Shearer, N. B. C. (2002). Loss of power within the nursing home zone. *Journal of Gerontological Nursing, 28*(1), 54–56.

Shearer, N. B. C., & Reed, P.G. (2004). Empowerment: Reformulation of a non-Rogerian concept. *Nursing Science Quarterly*, 17, 253–259.

Shearer, N. B. C. (2004). Relationships of contextual and relational factors to health empowerment in women. *Research and Theory for Nursing Practice, 18*, 357–370.

Shearer, N. B. C. (2007). Toward a nursing theory of health empowerment in homebound older women. *Journal of Gerontological Nursing, 33*(12), 38–45.

Shearer, N. B. C. (2009). Health empowerment theory as a guide for practice. *Geriatric Nursing, 30*(2, Suppl. 1), 4–10.

Shearer, N. B. C., & Fleury, J. (2006). Social support promoting health in older women. *Journal of Women & Aging, 18*(4), 3–17.

Shearer, N. B. C., Fleury, J., & Belyea, M. (2010). Randomized control trial of the health empowerment intervention. *Nursing Research, 59, 203–211. NIHMSID: 198546*

Shearer, N. B. C., Fleury, J., & Reed, P. G. (2009). The rhythm of health in older women with chronic illness. *Research and Theory for Nursing Practice, 23*, 148–160.

Sidani, S., & Braden, C. S. J. (1998). *Evaluating nursing interventions: A theory-driven approach.* Thousand Oaks, CA: Sage.

Walker, L. O., & Avant, K. C. (2005). *Strategies for theory construction in nursing* (4th ed.). Upper Saddle, NJ: Pearson/Prentice Hall.

Whittemore, R., & Grey, M. (2002). The systematic development of nursing interventions. *Journal of Nursing Scholarship, 34*(2), 115–120.

INTERLUDE III

Practitioner as Theorist: A Nurse's Toolkit for Theoretical Thinking

Pamela G. Reed

Inquiry is

> *a natural activity that is as intimately related to organic nature as the beating of a heart and the perches and flight of a bird....It arises from felt needs, employs both abstract and concrete tools, tests proposals in the laboratory of experience, and terminates in the resolution of the difficulties which occasioned that particular sequence of inquiry.* (Hickman, 2007, p. 37)

Thomas Kuhn's (1970/1962) *Structure of Scientific Revolutions* exploded into a controversy about scientific inquiry that continues into this century (Fuller, 2000). We know from writings of science historians, sociologists, and philosophers that the practice of science changes over time. Perspectives and strategies of knowledge development change as well. The focus of this column derives from an idea put forth 40 years ago by scholar Rosemary Ellis (1969), that of *practitioner as theorist*, as it may inspire a new path of theory development and expand the repertoire of strategies for knowledge production in nursing.

The current nursing shortage of practitioners and faculty has garnered nationwide attention. However, where there are shortages of nurses in practice and academia, there is also a shortage of nursing knowledge. Current statistics suggest that approximately 1% of nurses are developing knowledge for the remaining 99%. This is based on a survey of nurses' educational levels, along with a position statement by the American Association of Colleges of Nursing (2004) declaring that nurses with research doctorates are the knowledge producers for the discipline. The most

From P. G. Reed. (2008). Practitioner as theorist: A reprise. *Nursing Science Quarterly, 21,* pp. 315–321. Reprinted by permission of Sage Publications.

recent U.S. National Sample Survey of Registered Nurses indicates the following distribution of educational degrees among the nearly 3 million registered nurses in the United States: Doctorate in nursing or related field, 0.9%; Masters, 12%; Bachelor, 32%; Associate, 34%; and Diploma, 17.5%, with the remaining unknown (U.S. Department of Health and Human Resources & Health Resources and Services Administration [HRSA], 2004).

This same HRSA report indicated that the numbers of nurses in all higher educational programs are on the rise. The increase in practitioners and educational programs, particularly the Doctorate of Nursing Practice (DNP), presents a significant opportunity to expand the base of knowledge producers. Nursing practitioners are an untapped resource for generating nursing theories to enhance human well-being and health care.

MAKING PRACTITIONERS' THEORIZING EXPLICIT

The ability to theorize is a fundamental characteristic of human beings, the foundation of which is developed early in life and extends to the intentional activities of scientists (Ellis, 1969; Kaplan, 1964; Magnani, 2001; Vosniadou, 2001). Writings revealing the integrality of theory and practice and the potential for theory development among practitioners have intensified over the past decade. Fawcett and colleagues (Fawcett, Watson, Neuman, Walker, & Fitzpatrick, 2001) expanded the field of theorizing with their application of Carper's (1978) pluralistic paradigm of nursing knowledge. Doane and Varcoe (2005) fused theory and practice together in their concept of *compassionate action*. Chinn's (Chinn & Kramer, 2008) *praxis*, first discussed several years prior to this edition, denoted the transformative process of developing knowledge through critical practice. In addition, Reed and Lawrence (2008) proposed a paradigm for practice-based knowledge development in the clinical setting.

Theories and theorizing are embedded in practice, as many scholars have attested. An important next step is to address Ellis' (1969) original appeal to nursing to make practitioners' theorizing explicit. In her words,

> *If we really have a commitment to the future beyond the personal accumulation of wisdom from patient to patient, and if we wish to communicate this wisdom we must...have practitioners in nursing who are willing to be scholars as well and who have the interest, skill, and time to pursue the analyses and formulations [of nursing theories] and test them in practice.* (p. 1438)

Advancements in models of the nursing process have helped make more explicit the thinking strategies used in practice (see, for example, Pesut & Herman, 1999). However, these models typically focus on decision making, problem solving, critical thinking, or diagnostic and clinical reasoning. They do not focus on developing theory-based knowledge in practice—neither in terms of a methodology of theory development nor in terms of a substantive base of knowledge about human health processes. As Ellis (1969) pointed out, nurses may categorize assessment data, identify patterns, and form concepts, but they often stop short of advancing a theory by identifying links between concepts and outcomes of nursing care.

HISTORICAL TRENDS IN THEORY DEVELOPMENT

Nursing has a history of theory-development activities that have generated a diverse and dynamic structure of knowledge. Theoretical systems range from broad philosophic and paradigmatic statements, to conceptual models, middle-range theories, and theories that focus on specific practice situations. Approaches to developing nursing knowledge in the context of practice have changed over time and reflect changes in philosophies of science.

NIGHTINGALE AND EMPIRICISM

Florence Nightingale's 19th-century approach to theory development was influenced by British empiricism, which upheld the primacy of the five main senses in scientific knowledge. Her theorizing took the form of empirical generalizations, presented as canons in her *Notes on Nursing* (1859/1969). Nightingale worked horizontally on the empirical plane, using analogic reasoning to generalize across observations of patients and their environment, and then to organize specific statements about nursing and health. For example, from her observations of air, water, drainage, cleanliness, and light, she generalized statements about the *health of houses* and wrote a special section on that in her book.

Nightingale's theoretical statements were relational but not explanatory. She could *describe* a situation well and with her statistics predicted outcomes and reduced mortality rates. However, she did not have the conceptual tools to address health phenomena by explaining *how* or *why* environmental factors such as noise from the chattering hopes of visitors and music or the colors in varieties of flowers affected patient mood. That required theorizing vertically up to more abstract levels to access unseen (and therefore unaccepted) mystical concepts, such as sound and light waves, and psychological phenomena to explain a patient's well-being.

PEPLAU AND POST-POSITIVISM

Peplau's mid-20th-century approach to theorizing reflected postpositivist views dominant at the time, along with a dramatic shift from Nightingale's emphasis on *nursing as doing* to a focus on *nursing as knowing*. Peplau's theorizing allowed for abstract concepts and she applied her knowledge of interpersonal theories and underlying mechanisms, such as the psychodynamics of behavior and therapeutic milieu, to explain the healing power of nursing therapy. Her practice methodology centered on the nurse–patient relationship within a therapeutic environment. This was her context of knowledge production.

The corpus of Peplau's writings (see, for example, Peplau, 1988) presents a method of knowledge development that shifts between nursing practice and formal research. Peplau's *cycle of inquiry* (Reed, 1996) begins in the context of the nurse–patient relationship. The nurses' observations become the fundamental theoretical units, which are spiraled up drawing in relevant theories. Theoretical explanations are then *peeled out* from what the nurse has observed. The resulting theory is applied, tested, and transformed into nursing knowledge in the crucible of nursing practice.

ROGERS AND NEOMODERNISM

Theorizing in the 21st century reflects shifts in philosophy away from modernism toward postmodernism and post-postmodernism (or neomodernism) in which theories are no longer regarded as stable ideas that correspond to a higher truth but more as conceptual systems of ideas that influence and are influenced by their context. Although postmodernism decentered positivist and foundationalist notions of theory, theory nonetheless is still valorized as a prestigious activity across disciplines (Chaiklin, 2004).

Neomodern (Reed, 2006; Whall & Hicks, 2002) views reflected in theory development include the following: pluralism in sources of knowledge and methods of theory development; pragmatism balanced by assumptions about the mystery of life; belief in the capacity of human beings for innovation, agency, and well-being; an openness to change and critique; and valuing local truths as well as broader philosophies for their perspectives on what is emancipating, good, and healthful and other goals in nursing practice.

Rogerian thought (Rogers, 1970) is evident in the participatory and holistic perspectives underlying 21st-century nursing theorizing. Parse's (1987) *simultaneity* paradigm provides for nursing a discipline-defining alternative discourse to the medical model of health care: one that privileges patient perspectives and participation and values the nurse caregiver in knowledge production. Newman's *unitary-transformative* (UT) worldview (Newman, Sime, & Corcoran-Perry, 1991) identified substantive focuses for theory development such as the person's inherent potential for self-organization, innovative patterning, and connection to the environment. Cowling (2007) operationalizes Rogerian philosophy in his description of participatory action research, which united researchers, if not practitioners, and patients in the quest for nursing knowledge.

TOWARD PARTICIPATORY METHODS: AREAS FOR DIALOGUE

Theory building that includes the patient as partner (as well as the practicing nurse) equalizes the power between patients and nurses and fosters partnerships rather than paternalism in knowledge endeavors. The aim, as Barker (1999) warns in his discussion of nursing aspirations for professional status, is not "*to develop a professional, expert, and esoteric body of knowledge to be kept from, yet applied to the 'patient,'"* ...[this is] *"antithetical to the idea of partnership and reciprocity identified as the way forward in health care"* (p. 68).

It is time to reconsider assumptions about how knowledge development may occur and evaluate whether current methods align with our philosophies about nursing and science. There is need for dialogue and study on theory-development strategies that have fit and relevance in practice.

Questions for dialogue include the following:

- What traditional methods could be modified or reformulated as well as what new methods can be devised to better facilitate practitioner and patient involvement in knowledge development?
- What kind of participation do patients and families desire?
- What are the ethical considerations of practice-based theory development?
- Are practitioners interested in participating more actively in developing nursing knowledge?
- Do nurses care, as Peplau did, to *know* the why and how behind what they *do*?
- What resources are needed to do this in the practice setting?
- How can educational curricula support the learning needs of practitioners as knowledge producers?

EXTANT METHODS AND TOOLS OF CLINICAL INQUIRY

Several standard texts that target theory-development strategies are available in nursing, for example, Chinn and Kramer (2008), Walker and Avant (2005); and Reed and Shearer (2009). These texts include traditional strategies used by researchers as well as contemporary approaches relevant to practice settings. For example, Chinn and Kramer (2008) present a section on *practice-based evidence* whereby "evidence is generated out of, or situated in, the context from which it is generated" (p. 65); this kind of evidence may be preferable to that generated by top-down (research to practice) strategies, such as randomized clinical trials that strip away too much of the context relevant to nursing practice. In addition, texts on qualitative methods and on the practice and research methodologies of Parse's and Newman's nursing theories provide a wealth of ideas for practice-based theory-development strategies.

Methods and tools of clinical inquiry already exist that are potentially useful to practitioners in generating theory. These include grounded theory methodology, clinical reasoning, structured reflection, participatory action research, and clinical conceptual frameworks. *Grounded theory methodology* is flexible and can be adapted to practice situations (Glaser, 1978; J. Holton for B. Glaser, personal communication, June 6, 2008). It is a method grounded in patient caregiving processes, which include assessment and observation, organizing and interpreting data, identifying links and patterns in the data, and validating findings with the patient.

Pesut and Herman's (1999) comprehensive work in *clinical reasoning* has been applied in recent research (Kautz, Kuiper, Pesut, Knight-Brown, & Daneker, 2005) that extends scholarly work on critical thinking to study dimensions of clinical reasoning that may become tools for practice-based theory development. Rolfe and Gardner's (2005) *reflexive model of evidence-based practice* combines strategies of action research and Schön's (1983) reflection-in-action and single-case experimentation to form and test hypotheses relevant to nursing care in a specific patient care situation. Reed and Lawrence (2008) described structures called *clinical conceptual frameworks* as a mechanism for clinicians to transform interactions with patients and other data into theory form. The frameworks can be used to help clinicians articulate and formalize their personal theories and identify areas of inquiry in patient care.

NEW PERSPECTIVES

Less conventional tools and strategies for theorizing may evolve out of the dynamic context of nursing practice. New perspectives on theory development may be helpful in stimulating thinking on how to facilitate practice-based theory development and, as Ellis (1969) pleaded, make practitioner theories more explicit.

GUERRILLA THEORIZING

Guerrilla theorizing describes one perspective on how nurses in practice may engage in theory development. This concept, derived in part from the dynamic nature of nursing practice coupled with neomodern views from nursing and contemporary science, emphasizes participatory practices, the person–environment process of change, pragmatism and pluralism in knowledge building, and voices of patients and bedside caregivers in nursing theory and practice. The etymology of the term *guerrilla* indicates that the word means *small war*, the diminutive of the Spanish term for war, *Guerra*. The word originated in the early 1800s in reference to the Spanish resistance against Napoleon (Webster's, 1996). However, the term has come to have wide application as an adjective to describe strategies not of warfare but of bold and creative human endeavors including art, photography, marketing, graphic design, and even garage sales and an online physician group fighting back against the corporatization of health care.

Guerrilla-based strategies are unconventional, culturally sensitive, embedded or integrated in the local context, and dedicated to a human cause or mission. Smith's (2007) description of *guerrilla art* is analogous to nursing theorizing. Guerrilla art involves making something that is innovative, flexible, and impermanent, and which derives from the practitioner's inspiration and knowledge as well as out of ethical concern and interaction with one's immediate world. For the nurse, this refers to any of a variety of interactions with patients and their environment that can inform a theory. Furthermore, just as guerrilla art undergoes unique changes when exposed to the elements or is dampened by rain, so too can nurses' theories change in creative ways through their grounded practice with patients.

Practitioners' guerrilla theorizing also resembles what Carver (2002) labeled *theories in the wild* to describe knowledge that is produced in context, interpretive, partial, and always under construction. Carver's (2002) phrase fits the complex and sometimes messy context of nursing practice, where building knowledge is done *with* not just *for* patients and their families and includes the indigenous knowledge of those intimately involved in the health care experience. As Peirce (as cited in Hickman, 2007) expressed, science is not a static body of knowledge but the "concrete life of persons who are working to find out the truth" (p. 247).

Finally, three related concepts—bricoleur, improvisation, and abduction—elaborate on what is meant by *guerrilla theorizing*. They also provide a beginning infrastructure for practice-based theory development.

PRACTITIONER-THEORIST AS BRICOLEUR

Bricoleur is a French term referring to a person who constructs or creates objects or ideas (the *bricolage*) with what is at hand (Manser, 2002). Many sources cite anthropologist Lévi-Strauss' 1966 book, *The Savage Mind*, in describing the bricoleur: One who uses imagination as well as existing knowledge to piece together a diversity of raw materials, objects, methods, philosophies, or ideas that are *at hand* (as opposed to being accessed from outside one's immediate environment) in producing a coherent, new structure (conceptual or concrete) to address a problem. The bricoleur is often described in the context of discussions of qualitative or social research strategies (Denzin & Lincoln, 2003; Kincheloe, 2005).

In their classic description of a bricoleur theorist, Weinstein and Weinstein (1991) depict the bricoleur as one who engages in "disciplined conceptual play" and "seeks generality through particularity" (p. 161). Similarly, practice-based theories are constructed from the particular experiences of patient and nurse but are also *symbolic* constructions (Kaplan, 1964) that therefore reach out to a more general meaning beyond the data. Gobbi (2005) applied the term to describe the everyday work of nurses, as both intellectual and technical bricoleurs who adeptly cobble together a variety of elements at hand to formulate a theoretical framework for action. Thus, the unconventional, resourceful, action-oriented, synthetic approach of the bricoleur pertains to the nurse as both practitioner and theorist.

IMPROVISATION

Theory development in nursing practice shares a main characteristic, improvisation, with two unlike occupations, wildland firefighter and jazz musician. Improvisation involves creation of something out of preexisting elements, in the moment and in the natural setting. Weick's (2001) study of wildland firefighting and naturalistic decision making (NDM) demonstrated the importance of improvisation in NDM theorizing-in-action. Improvisation requires discipline and depth of experience as well as "unprogrammed" challenges. He also found that it was more effective to put forth loosely developed hunches than firm hypotheses (typically done in theorizing), which constrain creative thinking. Relevant to theorizing, Weick found that this form of thinking was understood more appropriately as a process of *sense making* than as decision making.

In reference to jazz, a story is told about the jazz musician and composer, Miles Davis, who was known for hiring very capable musicians. Just prior to a recording session, instead of handing out the standard charts of music, he gave each musician small pieces of paper and said, "This is your part." His intent was to create spontaneity yet have the musicians reach beyond themselves and the written music. His approach allowed for artistic freedom while adhering to rules of music theory. This combination of art and theory kept the performance fresh for musicians and audience while generating a cohesive sound.

Similarly, the practitioner scholar may be able to produce cohesive structures of knowledge called *theories* through a combination of rules of science and artful application of patterns of knowing in their work with patients. Just as improvisation involves balance between disciplinary rules and personal creativity, theory development is a science and an art.

ABDUCTIVE REASONING

The two widely known forms of logic, Aristotle's deductive syllogistic logic and Bacon's inductive logic, are insufficient for theory development. Abduction, a creative form of logic initially described by 20th-century philosopher of science Charles Peirce, plays an integral role in the discovery processes of theory development (Magnani, 2001; Yu, 2001). Abduction is a process of formulating plausible explanations from empirical observations and other knowledge sources. Abductive reasoning requires boldness and creativity. It is *ampliative* in that this form of reasoning expands beyond the information at hand. As theories "deal with ... entities that are invisible" (Yu, 2001, p. 281), they cannot posit ideas directly from the observed phenomena; guessing or taking conceptual leaps is required.

Abductive reasoning is found repeatedly in descriptions of thinking patterns that underlay theory-development strategies: For example, there is Popper's (1962/1965) concept of *conjecture* in putting forth theory testing ideas; Glaser's (1978) *conceptual leaps* deemed necessary in the discovery of grounded theory; and the process of *puzzling* (Lipshitz, 2001; Walsh, Moss, Lawless, McKelvie, & Duncan; 2008), which favors puzzle seeking over problem solving and employs action theory to develop knowledge in a professional practice.

Typically, abduction is described as useful in situations where knowledge and protocol are lacking and where solutions are neither clear-cut nor easily solved. More specifically, abduction is a strategy for producing new knowledge (theory), whereby the nurse applies creative insight and knowledge to generate and prioritize potential explanations for the problem at hand. With abduction, the experience or observation occurs first, followed by generation of hypotheses or potential explanations. To get beyond merely solving a problem and into theorizing, nurses need to entertain *why* something is or might be occurring or why an intervention works. Nursing science is about explaining as well as describing. Theories deliver in terms of providing scientific descriptions and explanations. Theories, within varying scopes, deliver on this.

Abduction is garnering increasing attention as a way of thinking theoretically in practice environments. In Kathryn Montgomery's (2006) book, *How Doctors Think*, the journalist promoted abductive thinking as the process underlying physicians' clinical judgment and theorizing for individual cases. Similarly, Hands (2001), as an economist, appropriated Peirce's abduction for his own profession, identifying it as an economics methodology. He stated that a good economist thinks abductively and posited that abductive inferences seem to be the "main 'stuff' of good science…[representing] the explanatory hunches and the creative insights that are the mainstay of successful scientific practice" and what is "truly novel and knowledge expanding about human inquiry" (p. 224). He also concludes that abduction may apply to other professions.

NETS OF NURSING KNOWLEDGE

Popper's (1934/1968) epigraph to his 1934 book, *The Logic of Scientific Discovery*, is a maxim by the 18th-century philosopher Novalis: "Theories are nets: only he who casts will catch" (p. 11). Popper elaborated later in his book: "Theories are nets cast to catch what we call 'the world': to rationalize, to explain, and to master it. We endeavour to make the mesh ever finer and finer" (p. 59). His statement reflected the significant influence of theories on translating our observations into meaning and action. However, there is another net metaphor that better represents how practitioners interact with theories today.

This net metaphor was inspired by a book about the roles of women in prehistory (Adovasio, Soffer, & Page, 2007). In one chapter, the authors describe life in Late Paleolithic society 26,000 years ago, where net hunting was a communal affair. The women constructed the nets on the run, adjusting the mesh bigger and smaller to accommodate the varying sizes of life forms available, from large mammals to birds and even insects. Unlike Popper's fishing net that is tossed out repeatedly and mechanically to catch and then master every bit of an unchanging reality, practice-based nursing theories are conceived to be more like the women's traveling nets, constructed on the go within a context and a community; and organic—capable of diversity and adaptation to the current situation, and evolving through interactions with the complex, changing environment.

Theories developed in action are more responsive to the changing needs of a situation. Weick's (2001) firefighter research revealed that *thinking in action* or thinking by taking action, in contrast to *thinking and acting*, was what produced effective knowledge. Magnani (2001) expanded his idea of theoretical abduction to emphasize *manipulative* abduction, *a thinking through doing* in contrast to thinking *about* doing (p. 309).

Action is a reality of practice. So, whereas practitioners may face added challenges in practice-based theory development, it may be found that their action orientation provides distinct advantages over traditional approaches to theorizing. "Scientific creativity is sharpened, not dulled, by rubbing against the whetstone of reality" (Raymo, 2006, p. 72).

QUESTIONS FOR REFLECTION

1. In thinking about your work in nursing, what experiences have you had that triggered a new idea you would like to pursue?
2. Of the various strategies in the article for thinking theoretically, which one best fits your style of thinking or working? Does this strategy help you balance "following the rules" with your "personal creativity" in building knowledge?
3. Does the notion of guerrilla theorizing relate to the way you link knowledge to your nursing practice?
4. How might guerrilla theorizing or other strategies be used in a research project?
5. Do you think that practicing nurses are interested in learning ways to develop knowledge and theories in practice? Are there barriers to doing this in practice? What resources would be helpful?

REFERENCES

Adovasio, J. M., Soffer, O., & Page, J. (2007). *The invisible sex: Uncovering the true rolls of women in prehistory*. New York: Smithsonian.

American Association of Colleges of Nursing. (2004). *Position statement on the practice doctorate in nursing*. Washington, DC: Author.

Barker, P. (1999). *The philosophy and practice of psychiatric nursing*. Edinburgh, UK: Churchill Livingstone.

Carper, B. A. (1978). Fundamental patterns of knowing in nursing. *Advances in Nursing Science, 1*, 13–23.

Carver, C. F. (2002). Structures of scientific theories. In P. Machamer & M. Silberstein (Eds.), *The Blackwell guide to the philosophy of science* (pp. 55–79). Malden, MA: Blackwell.

Chaiklin, H. (2004). Problem formulation, conceptualization, and theory development. In A. R. Roberts & K. R. Yeager (Eds.), *Evidence based practice manual: Research and outcome measures in health and human services* (pp. 95–101). New York: Oxford University Press.

Chinn, P. L., & Kramer, M. K. (2008.) *Integrated theory and knowledge development in nursing* (7th ed.). St. Louis, MO: Mosby.

Cowling, W. R. (2007). A unitary participatory vision of nursing knowledge. *Advances in Nursing Science, 30*, 61–70.

Denzin, N. K., & Lincoln, Y. S. (2003). *Collecting and interpreting qualitative materials* (2nd ed.). Thousand Oaks, CA: Sage.

Doane, G. H., & Varcoe, C. (2005). Toward compassionate action: Pragmatism and the inseparability of theory/practice. *Advances in Nursing Science, 28*, 81–90.

Ellis, R. (1969). Practitioner as theorist. *American Journal of Nursing, 69,* 1434–1438.

Fawcett, J., Watson, J., Neuman, B., Walker, P. H., & Fitzpatrick, J. J. (2001). On nursing theories and evidence. *Journal of Nursing Scholarship, 33,* 115–119.

Fuller, S. (2000). *Thomas Kuhn: A philosophical history of our times.* Chicago: University of Chicago Press.

Glaser, B. G. (1978). *Theoretical sensitivity.* Mill Valley, CA: Sociology Press.

Gobbi, M. (2005). Nursing practice as bricoleur activity: A concept explored. *Nursing Inquiry, 12,* 117–125.

Hands, D. W. (2001). *Reflection without rules: Economic methodology and contemporary science theory.* Edinburgh, UK: Cambridge University Press.

Hickman, L. A. (2007). *Pragmatism as post-postmodernism: Lessons from John Dewey.* New York: Fordham University Press.

Kaplan, A. (1964). *The conduct of inquiry: Methodology for behavioral science.* New York: Thomas Y. Crowell.

Kautz, D. D., Kuiper, R. A., Pesut, D. J., Knight-Brown, P., & Daneker, D. (2005). Promoting clinical reasoning in undergraduate nursing students: Application and evaluation of the outcome present state test (OPT) model of clinical reasoning. *International Journal of Nursing Education Scholarship, 2,* 1–21.

Kincheloe, J. L. (2005). On to the next level: Continuing the conceptualization of the bricolage. *Qualitative Inquiry, 11,* 323–350.

Kuhn, T. S. (1970). *The structure of scientific revolutions* (2nd ed.). Chicago: University of Chicago Press. (Original work published 1962)

Lévi-Strauss, C. (1966). *The savage mind.* Chicago: University of Chicago Press.

Lipshitz, R. (2001). Puzzle-seeking and model-building on the fire ground. In E. Salas & G. Klein (Eds.), *Linking expertise and naturalistic decision making* (pp. 337–345). Mahwah, NJ: Lawrence Erlbaum.

Magnani, L. (2001). Epistemic mediators and model-based discovery in science. In L. Magnani & N. J. Nersessian (Eds.), *Model-based reasoning: Science, technology, values* (pp. 305–329). New York: Kluwer Academic/Plenum.

Manser, J. H. (2002). *The facts on file dictionary of foreign words and phrases.* New York: Checkmark.

Montgomery, K. (2006). *How doctors think: Clinical judgment and the practice of medicine.* New York: Oxford University Press.

Newman, M. A., Sime, A. M., & Corcoran-Perry, S. A. (1991). The focus of the discipline of nursing. *Advances in Nursing Science, 14,* 1–6.

Nightingale, F. (1969). *Notes on nursing: What it is, and what it is not.* New York: Dover. (Original work published 1859)

Parse, R. R. (1987). *Nursing science: Major paradigms, theories, and critiques.* Philadelphia: W. B. Saunders.

Peplau, H. E. (1988). The art and science of nursing: Similarities, differences, and relations. *Nursing Science Quarterly, 1,* 8–15.

Pesut, D. J., & Herman, J. (1999). *Clinical reasoning the art and science of critical and creative thinking.* Albany, NY: Delmar.

Popper, K. R. (1965). *Conjectures and refutations: The growth of scientific knowledge.* New York: Harper Torchbooks. (Original work published 1962)

Popper, K. R. (1968). *The logic of scientific discovery.* New York: Harper Torchbooks. (Original work published 1934)

Raymo, C. (2006). *Walking zero: Discovering cosmic space and time along the prime meridian.* New York: Walker.

Reed, P. G. (1996). Transforming practice knowledge into nursing knowledge—A revisionist analysis of Peplau. *Journal of Nursing Scholarship, 28,* 29–33.

Reed, P. G. (2006). Neomodernism and evidence based nursing: Implications for the production of nursing knowledge. *Nursing Outlook, 54*(1), 36–38.

Reed, P. G., & Lawrence, L. A. (2008). A paradigm for the production of practice-based knowledge. *Journal of Nursing Management, 16,* 422–432.

Reed, P. G., & Shearer, N. B. C. (2009). *Perspectives on nursing theory* (5th ed.). Philadelphia: Wolters Kluwer/Lippincott Williams & Wilkins.

Rogers, M. E. (1970). *An introduction to the theoretical basis of nursing.* Philadelphia: F. A. Davis.

Rolfe, G., & Gardner, L. (2005). Towards a nursing science of the unique: Evidence, reflexivity and the study of persons. *Journal of Research in Nursing, 10,* 297–310.

Schön, D. A. (1983). *The reflective practitioner: How professionals think in action.* New York: Basic Books.

Smith, K. (2007). *Guerilla art kit: Everything you need to put your message out into the world.* New York: Princeton Architectural Press.

U.S. Department of Health and Human Resources & Health Resources and Services Administration. (2004). *The registered nurse population: Findings from the 2004 national sample survey of registered nurses.* Retrieved June 18, 2007, from http://bhpr.hrsa.gov/healthworkforce/rnsurvey04/

Vosniadou, S. (2001). Mental models in conceptual development. In L. Magnani & N. J. Nersessian (Eds.), *Model-based reasoning: Science, technology, values* (pp. 353–368). New York: Kluwer Academic/Plenum.

Walker, L. O., & Avant, K. C. (2005). *Strategies for theory construction in nursing* (4th ed.). Upper Saddle River, NJ: Pearson/Prentice Hall.

Walsh, K., Moss, C., Lawless, J., McKelvie, R., & Duncan, L. (2008). Puzzling practice: A strategy for working with clinical practice issues. *International Journal of Nursing Practice, 14,* 94–100.

Webster's new universal unabridged dictionary. (1996). New York: Barnes and Noble.

Weick, K. E. (2001). Tool retention and fatalities in wildland fire settings: Conceptualizing the naturalistic. In E. Salas & G. Klein (Eds.), *Linking expertise and naturalistic decision making* (pp. 321–336). Mahwah, NJ: Lawrence Erlbaum.

Weinstein, D., & Weinstein, M. A. (1991). Georg Simmel: Sociological bricoleur. *Theory, Culture & Society, 8,* 151–168.

Whall, A. L., & Hicks, F. D. (2002). The unrecognized paradigm shift in nursing: Implications, problems, and possibilities. *Nursing Outlook, 50,* 72–76.

Yu, Q. (2001). Model-based reasoning and similarity in the world. In L. Magnani & N. J. Nersessian (Eds.), *Model-based reasoning: Science, technology, values* (pp. 275–286). New York: Kluwer Academic/Plenum.

Clinical Scholarship: History and Future Possibilities

Elaine G. Jones

Scholarly inquiry historically has been housed in university settings with the main responsibility for research and other scholarly activities assigned to academicians (Schlotfeldt, 1992). However, clinical scholarship represents a perspective of scholarly inquiry that extends somewhat beyond the traditional practices of science. Understanding the historical context of clinical scholarship provides a foundation for discussing new ways to think about theory and knowledge development in nursing. In this chapter, I focus on the history of clinical scholarship in nursing, including a look at movements related to scholarship. I draw from historical perspectives and contemporary events to propose ideas for the future of clinical scholarship, particularly in reference to advanced practice nurses.

Reflecting on the evolution of clinical scholarship in nursing as well as reviewing the contemporary movements of evidence-based practice (EBP) and translational research may offer insights into ways that practicing nurses can be active participants in the development of nursing knowledge in the 21st century. Reviewing these areas also provide a context for proposing ideas for the future of clinical scholarship and how doctorally prepared nurses in practice will participate in knowledge development.

DEFINING TERMS

It is helpful to begin our exploration of nursing scholarship by defining a few key terms. The term *scholarship* is often used in publications as a noun without a definition. For example, Boyer (1996) spoke of "… clinical practice as a form of scholarship" (p. 1). Webster's *New World College Dictionary* (Neufeldt & Guralnik, 1996) defined scholarship (noun) as "the systematized knowledge of a learned person, exhibiting accuracy, critical ability, and thoroughness; erudition; the knowledge attained by scholars, collectively" (p. 1201). The definition of scholarship can be applied in nursing, as systematized knowledge attained by nursing scholars collectively. However, the definition does not address the process of knowledge development or the relationships between nursing knowledge, theories, research, and practice.

The term *scholarly* is typically used as an adjective, as in "scholarly inquiry," but the term is not defined. Again, the dictionary (Neufeldt & Guralnik, 1996) provided some clarity: "(adj.) 1) of or characteristic of a scholar; 2) having or showing much knowledge, accuracy, and critical ability; 3) devoted to learning; studious" (p. 1201). Furthermore, a *scholar* is defined as "a learned person; a specialist in a particular branch of learning ..." (p. 1201).

Perspectives about the links of practice to scientific knowledge have evolved over time as evident in the terms used to discuss nursing scholarship and practice (see Table 8.1). The definitions of some terms suggest that while nursing practice was considered a science-based practice, practice was not always regarded as an integral context for knowledge development. A question to ponder is to ask what practices of knowledge development are implied by the various terms, and how might advanced practice nurses engage in these forms of knowledge development to promote clinical scholarship today.

Nurses with doctorates have been leading scholars throughout the 20th century, encouraged to contribute to nursing knowledge through research and theory building. In contrast, nurses in practice have been encouraged to *utilize* the knowledge generated by nursing scholars to guide practice and to identify nursing problems for nursing scholars to study (e.g., Burns & Grove, 2003). The history of clinical nursing scholarship, beginning with Nightingale, belies the fact that practice was meant to be a key source not only of knowledge application but also of knowledge development.

NIGHTINGALE: NURSE EXEMPLAR OF SCHOLARSHIP

Florence Nightingale (1820–1910), founder of professional nursing, embodied nursing scholarship. She was a well-educated woman and consummate scholar. Many name her as the first nurse researcher (e.g., Burns & Grove, 2009; Kelly & Joel, 1996). Nightingale drew from her keen empirical observations, sense of moral commitment, and compilation of impressive statistics and other evidence to lead reform in care of the sick. She reformed health care of the British Army at Scutari to reduce the mortality rate from 42% to 2.2% and initiated a reform in nursing education with the establishment of the Nightingale Training School for nurses. She was adamant about the importance of careful, accurate observations as a basis for effective nursing care. In fact, she dedicated an entire chapter in her *Notes on Nursing* (Nightingale, 1859/1969) to the importance of accurate observations as the basis for effective patient care. For example, she wrote that

> it may safely be said, not that the habit of ready and correct observation will by itself make us useful nurses, but that without it we shall be useless with all our devotion. (Nightingale, 1859/1969, p. 63)

TABLE 8.1

Terms Used in Describing Relationships Between Nursing Theory, Research, and Practice

Term	Definition
Research	"Diligent, systematic inquiry or investigation to validate and refine existing knowledge and generate new knowledge" (Burns & Grove, 2009, p. 719).
Nursing research	"... a formal, systematic, and rigorous process of inquiry used to generate and test theories about the health-related experiences of human beings within their environments and about the actions and processes that nurses use in practice" (Fawcett & Garity, 2009, p. 5).
Research-based practice	A "systematic, rigorous, and precise way of translating research findings into practice" (Hamric, Spross, & Hanson, 2009, p. 141). (Note that the word *translate* is used here in its generic meaning, rather than the specific meaning in the term *translational research*, referring to the process of moving research findings into practice.)
Scholarship	"... the intellectual attainments that result from study and research in a particular field or branch of knowledge" (American Heritage Dictionary, 1985, p. 1098).
Clinical scholarship	1. "Knowledge derived from the analysis and synthesis of observations of clients and patients...a complex activity that has as its purpose the discovery, organization, analysis, synthesis, and transmission of knowledge resulting from client-oriented nursing practice" (Palmer, 1986, p. 318). 2. "... is an approach that enables evidence-based nursing and development of best practices to meet the needs of clients efficiently and effectively...requires the identification of desired outcomes; the use of systematic observation and scientifically-based methods to identify and solve clinical problems ..." (Sigma Theta Tau Clinical Scholarship Task Force, 1999b, p. 5). 3. "a professional value and intellectual process, grounded in curiosity about why our clients respond the way they do and why we, as nurses, do the things we do" (Dreher, 1999, p. 29). 4. Scholarship is "certain habits of mind" (Diers, 1995, p. 25); modifying the term *scholarship* with the word *clinical* highlights the observational or practice dimension of the scholarly activities, without diminishing the required intellectual rigor (Diers, 1995).
Scholarship of practice (application)	Research skills to test clinical knowledge and new practice strategies (American Association of Colleges of Nursing, 1999).
Evidence-based practice (EBP)	1. "... is the deliberate and critical use of theories about human beings' health-related experiences to guide actions associated with each step of the nursing process" (Fawcett & Garity, 2009, p. 8) broader than research utilization. 2. "... the integration of individual clinical expertise with the best available external clinical evidence from systematic research" (Sackett, Rosenberg, Gray, Haynes, & Richardson, 1996, p. 71). 3. [EBP] stresses use of research findings as well as other sources of credible facts, information or data (Stetler et al., 1998).
Translational research	1. research to apply scientific discoveries in practical applications, in order to improve human health (NINR, 2010). 2. "A study of how research knowledge that is directly or indirectly relevant to health behavior eventually serves the public" (Sussman, Valente, Rohrbach, Skara, & Pentz, 2006, p. 9). May be guided by theories such as diffusion of innovation (Rogers, 2003).

Her emphasis on meticulous observations parallels the emphasis on precise measurement and systematic data collection in contemporary science and nursing research. She reminded readers that the goal of observation (data collection) was to improve care:

> In dwelling upon the vital importance of *sound* observation, it must never be lost sight of what observation is for. It is not for the sake of piling up miscellaneous information or curious facts, but for the sake of saving life and increasing health and comfort. (Nightingale, 1859/1969, p. 70)

Despite this emphasis on empirical observation, however, Nightingale also employed critical and theoretical thinking. By this, she formulated empirical generalizations about the data she gathered. The chapter, titles in her *Notes on Nursing*, can be viewed as a list of some of her major empirical generalizations that provide knowledge for practice in specific areas of nursing care (Reed & Zurakowski, 1996). In particular, Nightingale (1859/1969) advanced theoretical ideas about the relationship of physical and social environmental factors to human health.

Nightingale's words echo ongoing reminders that the goal of clinical observations and nursing scholarship is to build nursing knowledge for improved nursing practice and optimal patient outcomes (Munro, 1997; National Institute of Nursing Research [NINR], 2010). Nightingale's (1859/1969) theories about effective nursing care were detailed in her writings. For example, she wrote that there are five essential points in securing the health of houses: pure air, pure water, efficient drainage, cleanliness, and light. She proposed an inverse relationship between the health of the house and the health of the inhabitants: "Without these (5 concepts), no house can be healthy. And it will be unhealthy just in proportion as they are deficient" (p. 15). Her theory about the relationship between the condition of the house and the health of its inhabitants provided an organizational framework for directing effective nursing care for the sick. These ideas were the predecessors of what were to become two key concepts in nursing's metaparadigm: *environment* and *health*.

Major events regarding nursing knowledge development continued in the 100 years following publication of *Notes on Nursing*, as listed in Table 8.2. The list of selected events reveals that disciplinary changes in research and theory practices occurred relatively independent of each other. The turn of the 20th century brought an increased focus on nursing practice as a source for generating nursing knowledge as well as for applying theory and other forms of knowledge. The importance of scientific knowledge in providing nursing care is a professional legacy that continues on into contemporary nursing (Fawcett & Garity, 2009).

THE EVOLUTION OF CLINICAL SCHOLARSHIP

The term *clinical scholarship* appeared in nursing literature more than 20 years ago to address the intimate relationship between theory, research, scholarship, and practice. Palmer (1986) emphasized the inductive nature of clinical scholarship and

TABLE 8.2

Selected Research and Theory Events in Nursing Knowledge Development

Year	Key Event
1869	Nightingale publishes *Notes on Nursing: What it is and what it is not* (Nightingale, 1859/1969)
1922	Sigma Theta Tau was founded; a community of nursing scholars (www.nursingsociety.org)
1955	The American Nurses Foundation was founded to fund nursing research (www.anfonline.org)
1950–1960s	Early nursing theorists from Columbia University Teacher's College (including Peplau, Henderson, Hall, Abdellah, King, Wiedenbach) publish their works
1965	American Nurses' Association identified theory development as a significant goal (Meleis, 2007)
1968	First Nurse Scientist Conference on *The Nature of Science in Nursing* (Meleis, 2007)
1970s	Second-generation nursing theorists publish their works (including Rogers, Roy, King, Orem, Neuman), regarded as classic nursing conceptual models (see, for example, Fitzpatrick & Whall, 1996)
1975	Nursing Theories Conference Group (Meleis, 2007)
1980s	Marked increases in publications focusing on philosophy and theory development and criteria for the critique of extant nursing conceptual models and theories (Nicoll, 1986)
1983	*Image: The Journal of Nursing Scholarship* inaugurated the theme of clinical scholarship with Associate Editor Donna Diers (www.wiley.com/bw/journal.asp?ref=1527–6546 or www.nursingsociety.org)
1986	The National Center for Nursing Research (NCNR) established (www.nih.gov/ninr)
1990s	Mid-range theories are distinguished from grand theories (Fawcett, 1993) and there is a marked increase in development of mid-range nursing theories (e.g., Smith & Liehr, 2003)
1992	The NCNR became the National Institute of Nursing Research (www.nih.gov/ninr)
2000	Noted increase in attention to the role of practice in knowledge development (Parker & Smith, 2010)

its use in improving patient care (Table 8.1). Schlotfeldt (1992) believed that professional nursing depended on clinical scholarship to "generate promising theories for testing that will advance nursing knowledge and insure nursing's continued essential services to humankind" (p. 8). Diers (1995) described scholarship as "certain habits of mind" (p. 25) and said that modifying the term *scholarship* with the word *clinical* highlighted the observational or practice dimension of the scholarly activities without diminishing the intellectual rigor required.

In 1997, Munro introduced a new format in the nursing journal, *Clinical Nurse Specialist*, emphasizing a closer relationship between research and practice, as clinical scholarship. Munro (1997) wrote that

> I am very excited about the new format of this Journal because research studies will no longer be in a separate section, but incorporated under the relevant heading. This

emphasizes the need to view clinical scholarship as basic to excellence in advanced practice. (p. 108)

The implication was that clinical scholarship is the work of nurse researchers and perhaps advanced practice nurses. However, the most important event in promoting clinical scholarship was the presentation of a white paper on clinical scholarship by Sigma Theta Tau International (STTI) at the 35th Biennial Convention (Sigma Theta Tau Clinical Task Force, 1999a). This paper is now published online as a resource paper (Sigma Theta Tau Clinical Task Force, 1999b).

THE SIGMA THETA TAU WHITE PAPER ON CLINICAL SCHOLARSHIP

The board of directors for STTI convened a task force on clinical scholarship serving from 1995 to 1997. The task force continued from 1997 to 1999 with new members, culminating in presentation of a white paper on clinical scholarship at the 35th Biennial Convention. The paper was grounded in the belief that "practice itself is a scholarly undertaking" (Sigma Theta Tau Clinical Scholarship Task Force, 1999a, p. 4) and calling for a closer relationship between practice and research. Clinical scholarship was defined as

> an approach that enables evidence-based nursing and development of best practices to meet the needs of clients efficiently and effectively. It requires the identification of desired outcomes; the use of systematic observation and scientifically-based methods to identify and solve clinical problems. (Sigma Theta Tau Clinical Scholarship Task Force, 1999a, p. 5)

The White Paper included exemplars of collaborations between academicians and practitioners to address clinical problems in diverse nursing care settings. Clinical scholarship was conceptualized as a means for achieving EBP, and so research and other evidence was used in deciding how to improve practice. However, this initial definition did not explicitly address the role of theory in scholarly practice. In some exemplars, the theoretical basis for the project was identified, and in other cases, there was no clear indication of a theoretical foundation. One exemplar of theory-based clinical scholarship presented in the STTI White Paper was Friedrich and Dreher's (1999) application of grief theory in a collaborative project between the University of Iowa Hospitals and Clinics and the College of Nursing to study adaptation to severe mental illness. The goal of the project was to improve outcomes for families caring for a family member with mental illness. Researchers and clinicians employed the theory in developing family-centered interventions and in the implementation and evaluation of a new family care model in practice.

CLINICAL SCHOLARSHIP IN PRACTICE

Following the Sigma Theta Tau White Paper, calls for clinical scholarship echoed in every aspect of nursing practice and education. Bell (2003) asked, "Where are the voices from practice who can describe innovative family interventions?" (p. 127).

Bell was adamant in her support for clinical scholarship as synthesis of practice knowledge and potential for contribution to theory building in family nursing. She believed that clinical scholarship required concurrent immersion in practice and analysis of the practice itself. She proposed use of Wright and Leahey's (2000) framework for clinical scholarship with distinctions between perceptual (observations), conceptual (analysis), and executive (taking action) skills. Bell (2003) reported using this framework in teaching clinical scholarship for graduate nursing students.

Bell distinguished between clinical research and clinical scholarship, as she called for greater participation in clinical scholarship by practitioners themselves. She described the process of *clinical research* as beginning with the researcher understanding a phenomenon, next describing it, and eventually designing and testing interventions. In contrast, she described *clinical scholarship* as beginning with examination of the current practice, next synthesizing practice knowledge (from diverse sources), and including making changes in a theory based on practice (Bell, 2003). She believed clinical scholarship was more complex than nursing research, as it "requires an immersion in clinical practice while simultaneously finding ways to articulate, describe, and analyze what is occurring within clinical practice" (Bell, 2003, p. 128). From her perspective, nurses in practice were essential for the process of clinical scholarship to occur.

CLINICAL SCHOLARSHIP IN NURSING EDUCATION

Scholarship of Students

Nursing educators began to find innovative ways to incorporate learning activities to promote clinical scholarship among their students. For example, Pullen, Reed, and Oslar (2001) reported that faculty created a capstone scholarly paper rather than a comprehensive nursing care plan in response to the emerging importance of clinical scholarship. They adopted Dreher's (1999) definition of clinical scholarship as "a professional value and intellectual process, grounded in curiosity about why our clients respond the way they do and why we, as nurses, do the things we do" (as cited in Pullen et al., 2001, p. 1). The authors posited that scholarly writing was an important foundation for clinical scholarship. Students received detailed instructions and mentoring for conducting a review of literature, synthesizing findings, and clinical reasoning, culminating in a capstone scholarly paper addressing holistic care of a patient.

Scholarship of Faculty

The American Association of Colleges of Nursing (AACN) published definitions of scholarship for the discipline of nursing in the same year (1999) that STTI published their white paper on clinical scholarship. The AACN (1999) defined *scholarship in nursing* as

> Those activities that systematically advance the teaching, research and practice of nursing through rigorous inquiry that 1) is significant to the profession 2) is creative,

3) can be documented, 4) can be replicated or elaborated, and 5) can be peer-reviewed through various methods. (p. 3)

The AACN 1999 document (p. 3) incorporated Boyer's (1990) four areas of scholarship in academic work:

1. Scholarship of discovery: where new and unique knowledge is generated
2. Scholarship of teaching: where the teacher creatively builds bridges between his or her own understanding and the students' learning
3. Scholarship of application: where the emphasis is on the use of new knowledge in solving society's problems
4. Scholarship of integration: where new relationships among disciplines are discovered (Boyer, 1990).

Examples of the *scholarship of discovery* included primary empirical research, historical research, theory development and testing, methodological studies, and philosophical inquiry and analysis. The scholarship of discovery was documented through peer-reviewed publications, presentations, grant awards, and mentorship.

Examples of the *scholarship of teaching* included development of innovative teaching and evaluation methods, program development, learning outcome evaluation, and professional role modeling. The scholarship of teaching was documented in peer-reviewed publications as well as published textbooks, presentations, and recognition as a master teacher (AACN, 1999).

The *scholarship of practice* encompassed all aspects of the delivery of nursing service and focused on the advancement of clinical knowledge in the discipline. Components of scholarship of practice included development of clinical knowledge, professional development, application of technical or research skills, and scholarly service such as development of practice standards. Documentation of scholarship of practice included peer-review publications, presentations related to practice, grant awards, and recognition as a master practitioner (AACN, 1999). This category of scholarship corresponded most closely to nurses' conceptualizations of clinical scholarship.

Examples of the *scholarship of integration* included activities such as integrative reviews of literature, analyses of health policy, and development of interdisciplinary education programs. Integration could also refer to interdisciplinary inquiry. Documentation was similar to documentation of other areas of scholarship, especially publication in peer-reviewed journals (AACN, 1999).

PROMOTING CLINICAL SCHOLARSHIP IN FACULTY

Faculty in university settings have been expected to engage in research and scholarship throughout academic history. The AACN did not delimit scholarship activities to doctorally prepared nursing faculty. However, many master's-prepared nursing faculty teaching in undergraduate programs were not expected to engage in research or scholarship. Jones and Van Ort (2001) believed that all nursing faculty were leaders in professional nursing and role models of scholarly practice for nursing students and therefore should be engaged in scholarship. These faculty were responsible for teaching students the importance of clinical scholarship and EBP, though they typically had little opportunity to engage in scholarly activities themselves. This lack of opportunity for scholarly pursuits, nontenure track notwithstanding, limits resources for personal fulfillment, academic achievement, and promotion in rank.

Jones and Van Ort (2001) proposed a model that has relevance today for strengthening organizational support for scholarship among clinical faculty, integrating scholarship with their other role responsibilities. According to the model, a faculty workgroup created a synthesized definition of clinical scholarship, which was the basis for evaluating faculty for promotion. Promotion criteria were revised to require documentation of clinical scholarship for promotion to the highest rank in the nontenure ranks. The definition of clinical scholarship was expanded beyond that of discovery to also include the areas of teaching, practice or integration, consistent with Boyer's (1990) and the AACN (1999) definitions. Van Ort, who was then dean of The University of Arizona College of Nursing, created a position for director of clinical scholarship (DCS; Dr. Jones) positioned within the Office of Nursing Research.

The DCS was responsible for mentoring and supporting clinical track (nontenure) faculty as they developed their scholarship ideas and projects. The DCS initiated individual appointments with each faculty to discuss areas of interest, created scholarship teams, and conducted writing groups for manuscripts and grant applications for funding to support scholarship activities. An example of scholarship of teaching conducted by nontenure eligible faculty under this model was evaluation of a student assignment, using a wellness contract as an effective method for teaching critical thinking (Feingold & Perlich, 1999). An example of scholarship of practice under this model was a faculty (Laura McRee) project "to evaluate the effectiveness of preoperative massage and music on the postoperative pain experience" (Jones & Van Ort, 2001, p. 144).

Administrative support is a key element in allocating the necessary fiscal and physical resources as well as faculty role expectations and rewards to promote clinical scholarship in faculty. Faculty practice plans should incorporate support for clinical scholarship as well as for clinical practice.

MOVEMENTS RELATED TO CLINICAL SCHOLARSHIP

Evidence-Based Practice

The term *EBP* has been in wide usage for nearly 20 years and is considered the desired outcome for clinical scholarship activities (Sigma Theta Tau Clinical Scholarship Task Force, 1999b). Sackett, Rosenberg, Gray, Haynes, and Richardson (1996) described EBP as the process of integrating individual clinical expertise with the best available external clinical evidence from systematic research and patient-based data and values. EBP differs from "research utilization" in that EBP incorporates the use of more and diverse knowledge sources—including data from the current clinical context rather than limiting the clinician to findings from a given study in determining best practices.

Efforts to achieve EBP address many issues related to clinical scholarship but do not always explicitly integrate theory in the process. Practitioners learn to critique research and to incorporate other sources of evidence in determining best practices in clinical care. For example, Rosswurm and Larrabee (1999) published a model for change to EBP, supporting a paradigm shift from tradition and intuition-driven practice to EBP. They noted that this paradigm shift was possible because nurses could access research findings far more easily (such as by the Internet) than in past years but that nurses still had difficulty synthesizing evidence and integrating their work into practice.

The process for implementing EBP is not unlike the research process, as it entails assessing and identifying the need for change, reviewing and critiquing available evidence to decide whether and what change in practice is warranted, if warranted implementing the practice based on the evidence, and then evaluating the new practice. However, although the decision to implement a certain practice is based on results of research, these decisions may not have an explicit theoretical basis. The authors said that "the selection of potential interventions and patient outcomes are based primarily on clinical judgment and system priorities and resources" (Rosswurm & Larrabee, 1999, p. 321). The participants used a worksheet to evaluate relevant research reports, culminating with an evidence-rating scale for each article. The worksheet did not include identification of the theoretical basis of the research. However, participants did identify relevant "process variables" as a result of synthesizing evidence, which may have represented implicit theoretical ideas in linking the proposed intervention with the desired patient outcomes.

Mohide and Coker (2005) also wrote about an organizational strategy for moving nurses toward more EBP. They viewed EBP as the *means* for shifting nursing culture toward clinical scholarship, rather than EBP as an *outcome* of clinical scholarship. The emphasis was on organizational support for an evidence-based nursing (EBN) committee, partnerships with academic nursing colleagues, and committee membership and activities. One of the first tasks of the EBN committee was to reach consensus about the concepts for EBP and identify a conceptual model for implementing change. There was careful attention to mentoring nurses in the process of EBP and evaluating research findings, but there was no mention of identifying the theoretical foundations for practice changes.

For EBP to promote nursing scholarship, this movement must more deliberately incorporate theory into the process. The theoretical dimensions of knowledge development are integral to all phases of EBP including conceptualizing the problem and determining what are effective and ethical approaches to addressing the problem.

Translational Research

Translational research focuses on promoting timely application of well-supported research findings in clinical settings. Sussman, Valente, Rohrbach, Skara, and Pentz

(2006) present several definitions of the term *translation* and clarify that "in the health professions [including nursing], *translation* describes an extended process of how research knowledge that is directly or indirectly relevant to health behavior eventually serves the public" (p. 9). The authors review models of how research may progress from basic research to dissemination for use in practice and describe barriers to achieving translation of research into practice. They identified one barrier as the historic professional distance between researchers and clinicians, with no clear research base for understanding why. "At present, it may take as long as one or two decades for original research" to be translated into routine (p. 8).

The authors provided recommendations for additional translational research to address this problem, for example, "determining which methods are most effective, cost-effective, and/or sustainable in assisting providers to stay abreast of the most recent scientific evidence in their areas of clinical specialization" (Sussman et al., 2006, p. 25) and which factors motivate them or serve as barriers to their use of that evidence in their clinical decision making. They emphasized that transdiscipline communication will be key to achieving EBP, with synergy between researchers and clinicians evaluating innovations with participation by health professionals in both academic and clinical settings.

Translational research focuses on identifying effective means of integrating extant knowledge from research to better understand facilitators and barriers of practices that improve health and well-being. The clinical scholarship of translational research may benefit the process through a more deliberate use of theory in the research method. Theory is the means by which data are translated into ideas for research and a structure for communicating and then testing these practice applications.

DNPS AND THE FUTURE OF CLINICAL NURSING SCHOLARSHIP

Most discussions of research or clinical scholarship cast nurses with Doctor of Philosophy (PhD) degrees as leaders in knowledge development and suggest that the role of nurses in practice—even those with practice doctorates such as the DNP—is to evaluate the merits of research findings for application in practice settings or to suggest areas for research.

Mundinger, Starck, Hathaway, Shaver, and Woods (2009) published a discussion by members of the Council for the Advancement of Comprehensive Care (CACC) about emerging programs offering a doctorate in nursing practice and the importance of building clinical scholarship. The CACC was formed in 2000 and members are deans of academic health center nursing schools and health policy experts from medicine and related fields. This council published a set of doctoral competencies for clinical doctoral education in 2006. The DNP competencies did not include "clinical scholarship," although the 11th competency indirectly addressed clinical scholarship relevant to EBP outcomes: "Use and synthesize evidence from practice and patient databases and analyze data to generate evidence from practice to improve patient care" (p. 70).

The CACC members who were establishing DNP programs discussed the importance of faculty's vision for clinical scholarship and described the importance of building a "culture of clinical scholarship" (p. 71) for a clinical doctorate. The primary means for establishing a culture of clinical scholarship was having an active faculty practice plan in place. This attention to faculty practice is consistent with other discussions about the importance of immersion in practice as a requisite of clinical scholarship.

Mundinger et al. (2009) said that "the cornerstone of clinical scholarship is the translation of best evidence into practice and guiding DNP students as they lead these efforts" (p. 73). They believed that all faculty needed to understand the importance and value of practice inquiry and its relationship to translational science and EBP. The clinician scholar's work might also seed other theory-building scholarship or impact policy. For example, a "methodical review of their clinical encounters could yield themes of patient care outcomes suitable to further research or a change in treatment policy" (p. 73).

PRACTICE INQUIRY: AN EXAMPLE OF CLINICAL SCHOLARSHIP IN ADVANCED PRACTICE

The University of Arizona DNP program culminates in a practice inquiry, which comprises a variety of research approaches, including those involved "a translation of research evidence into practice, evaluation of practice, improvement of the safety or quality of health care practice and outcomes, or participation in collaborative research" (DePalma & McGuire, 2005, p. 257). The practice inquiry embodies the student's synthesis of theory, research, and other evidence to address a clinical problem in advanced practice (University of Arizona College of Nursing, 2010).

One example of a practice inquiry designed to evaluate advanced practice was conducted by Thal (2010) and titled "Use of Standards of Care by Nurse Practitioners in Providing Care to Adolescents With Asthma at an Academic Nurse Managed Primary Care Clinic." Thal conducted a comprehensive review of research and other evidence and chose diffusion of innovation as the primary theory to inform her research. The purpose of her study was to evaluate the nature and extent to which nurses used standards of care with adolescents with asthma. She used a mixed-methods design to conduct a process evaluation. Thal reviewed 54 electronic records of patient visits at a nurse-managed school clinic. She also administered surveys and conducted interviews with eight nurse practitioners, many of whom were in academic as well as practice positions.

Data analysis revealed strong support for adopting best practice guidelines for care of adolescents with asthma from the National Heart Lung and Blood Institute (2007). However, documentation in the electronic charts did not reflect consistent implementation of the standards of care. Thal (2010) interpreted her results within the context of the diffusion of innovation theory to develop theory-based recommendations for improving care of adolescents with asthma and for continuing evaluations of advanced practice. Thal's (2010) practice inquiry provided an example of theory-based clinical scholarship in advanced practice.

The benefits of collaboration between nursing scientists, theorists, and practitioners to build nursing knowledge have been recognized for decades. However, full partnership between nurse clinicians—especially advanced practice nurses—and nurse scientists in knowledge and theory development have not been realized. Advanced practice nurses prepared at the doctoral level, such as the DNP nurse, will be key participants in using the methods of EBP and translational science, along with other methods yet to emerge. Fuller participation of practicing nurses in knowledge development can enhance the discipline's potential for clinical scholarship and development of innovations for practice.

THE FUTURE OF PRACTICE AND CLINICAL SCHOLARSHIP

New publications on clinical scholarship continue to appear as we strive to understand conceptualizations important to knowledge development in nursing and to articulate our theoretical views and philosophical foundations. New terms with similar definitions continue to appear in contemporary literature (Stillwell, Fineout-Overholt, Melnyk, & Williamson, 2010). Knowledge development will continue to be relevant, albeit referred to by different words. For example, the National Institutes of Health (e.g., NINR, 2010) advocate for more translational research to apply scientific discoveries into practical applications to improve human health, noting that this is really a "two-way street" between scientists and clinicians. This is reminiscent of the exemplars of academic–clinical collaborations presented in the STTI White Paper on Clinical Scholarship in 1999 and the collaborations presented in other reports about improving practice (e.g., Mohide & Coker, 2005). The importance of partnerships between nurses in academic settings and those in practice settings is often touted as an essential element in clinical scholarship. The potential for theory development through an iterative process within this relationship has not been realized (Higgins & Moore, 2004; Newman, 1972; Stetler et al., 1998).

Still relevant today, DeKeyser and Medoff-Cooper (2001) stated simply that "the basis of all nursing endeavors, including practice and research, lies in theory" (p. 329), with theory representing creative and coherent structures of nursing knowledge useful for practice. This applies to clinical scholarship endeavors as well. Yet, in publications about clinical scholarship, particularly in the EBP and TR literature, there is little mention of theory as an important part of the process of knowledge development for practice. We seem to have lost sight of Florence Nightingale's original practice of clinical scholarship, which generated publications of theoretical formulations relevant to practice. Through her synthesis of careful and systematic observations, theoretical compilation, esthetic practice of patient care, and an ethical commitment to improving human well-being, Nightingale advanced nursing to a scholarly profession.

Revisioning theory development based on new methods of inquiry in practice is needed, to open new pathways for practicing nurses to participate in knowledge development. For example, the idea of a practice inquiry may be developed by which practicing nurses derive and test theoretical ideas in practice. The movement toward preparing more practicing nurses with academic degrees at the doctoral level, DNP as well as PhD, is a distinct opportunity to advance knowledge-development efforts through clinical nursing scholarship. Advanced practice nurses who maintain an active practice while participating fully in academic life embody clinical scholarship through the synergy between practice, research, and theory in advancing nursing knowledge.

QUESTIONS FOR REFLECTION

1. What unique roles may practicing nurses have in nursing scholarship and knowledge development?
2. How might clinical nursing scholarship enhance evidence-based practice (EBP) beyond what EBP is commonly understood to be?
3. How might translational research be used to promote clinical nursing scholarship?
4. How can nursing students best learn clinical scholarship and participate in building nursing knowledge?

REFERENCES

American Association of Colleges of Nursing. (1999, March). *Defining scholarship for the discipline of nursing.* Washington, DC: Author.

American heritage dictionary (2nd college ed.). (1985). Boston: Houghton Mifflin.

Bell, J. M. (2003). Clinical scholarship in family nursing (editorial). *Journal of Family Nursing, 9*(2), 127–129.

Boyer, E. L. (1990). *Scholarship reconsidered: Priorities of the professoriate.* Princeton, NJ: Carnegie Foundation for the Advancement of Teaching.

Boyer, E. L. (1996). Clinical practice as scholarship. *Holistic Nursing Practice, 10*(3), 1–6.

Burns, N., & Grove, S. K. (2003). *Understanding nursing research* (4th ed.). St. Louis, MO: Saunders-Elsevier.

Burns, N., & Grove, S. K. (2009). *The practice of nursing research* (6th ed.). St. Louis, MO: Saunders-Elsevier.

DeKeyser, F. G., & Medoff-Cooper, B. (2001). A non-theorist's perspective on nursing theory: Issues of the 1990s. *Scholarly Inquiry for Nursing Practice: An International Journal, 15,* 329–341.

DePalma, J. A., & McGuire, D. G. (2005). Research. In A. B. Hamric, J. A. Spross, & C. Hanson (Eds.), *Advanced practice nursing: An integrative approach* (3rd ed., pp. 257–300). Philadelphia: Elsevier Saunders.

Diers, D. (1995). Clinical scholarship. *Journal of Professional Nursing, 11,* 24–30.

Dreher, M. C. (1999). Clinical scholarship: Nursing practice as an intellectual endeavor. In Sigma Theta Tau Clinical Scholarship Task Force (Ed.), *Clinical scholarship resource paper* (pp. 26–33). Retrieved December 4, 2010, from http://www.nursingsociety.org/aboutus/PositionPapers/Documents/clinical_scholarship_paper.pdf

Fawcett, J. (1993). *Analysis and evaluation of nursing theories.* Philadelphia: F. A. Davis.

Fawcett, J., & Garity, J. (2009). *Evaluating research for evidence-based nursing practice.* Philadelphia: F. A. Davis.

Feingold, C., & Perlich, L. J. (1999). Teaching critical thinking through a health-promotion contract. *Nurse Educator, 24,* 42–44.

Fitzpatrick, J., & Whall, A. (Eds.). (1996). *Conceptual models of nursing: Analysis and application* (3rd ed.). Stanford, CT: Appleton & Lange.

Friedrich, R. M., & Dreher, M. (1999). Clinical scholarship exemplar: The University of Iowa. In Sigma Theta Tau Clinical Scholarship Task Force (Ed.), *Clinical scholarship resource paper* (pp. 5–6). Retrieved December 4, 2010, from http://www.nursingsociety.org/aboutus/PositionPapers/Documents/clinical_scholarship_paper.pdf

Hamric, A. B., Spross, J. A., & Hanson, C. M. (2009). *Advanced practice nursing: An integrative approach.* St. Louis, MO: Saunders Elsevier.

Higgins, P. A., & Moore, S. M. (2004). Levels of theoretical thinking in nursing. In P. G. Reed, N. C. Shearer, & L. H. Nicoll (Eds.), *Perspectives on nursing theory* (4th ed., pp. 55–62). Philadelphia: Lippincott Williams, & Wilkins.

Jones, E. G., & Van Ort, S. (2001). Facilitating scholarship among clinical faculty. *Journal of Professional Nursing, 17*(3), 141–146.

Kelly, L. Y., & Joel, L. A. (1996). *The nursing experience: Trends, challenges, and transitions* (3rd ed.). New York: McGraw-Hill.

Meleis, A. I. (2007). *Theoretical nursing: Development and progress* (4th ed.). Philadelphia: Lippincott Williams, & Wilkins.

Mohide, E. A., & Coker, E. (2005). Toward clinical scholarship: Promoting evidence-based practice in the clinical setting. *Journal of Professional Nursing, 21,* 372–379.

Mundinger, M. O., Starck, P., Hathaway, D., Shaver, J., & Woods, N. F. (2009). The ABCs of the doctor of nursing practice: Assessing resources, building a culture of clinical scholarship, curricular models. *Journal of Professional Nursing, 25*(2), 69–74.

Munro, B. H. (1997). Improving nursing practice through clinical nursing scholarship. *Clinical Nurse Specialist, 11*(3), 108.

National Heart, Lung, and Blood Institute. (2007). *Expert Panel Report 3: Guidelines for the diagnosis and management of asthma* (NIH Publication No. 07–4051). Retrieved December 4, 2010, from http://www.nhlbi.nih.gov/guidelines/asthma/asthgdln.pdf

National Institute of Nursing Research. (2010). *NINR strategic plan.* Retrieved December 4, 2010, from http://www.ninr.nih.gov/NR/rdonlyres/9021E5EB-B2BA-47EA-B5DB-1-E4DB11B1289/4894/NINR_StrategicPlanWebsite.pdf

Neufeldt, V., & Guralnik, D. B. (Eds.). (1996). *Webster's new world college dictionary* (3rd ed.). New York: Simon & Schuster.

Newman, M. (1972). Nursing's theoretical evolution. In P. G. Reed, N. C. Shearer, & L. H. Nicoll (Eds.), *Perspectives on nursing theory* (4th ed., pp. 113–120). Philadelphia: Lippincott Williams, & Wilkins.

Nicoll, L. H. (Ed.). (1986). *Perspectives on nursing theory.* Boston: Little, Brown.

Nightingale, F. (1969). *Notes on nursing: What it is and what it is not.* New York: Dover. (Original work published 1859)

Palmer, I. S. (1986). The emergence of clinical scholarship a professional imperative. *Journal of Professional Nursing, 2,* 318–325.

Parker, M. E., & Smith, M. C. (2010). *Nursing theories & nursing practice* (3rd ed.). Philadelphia: F. A. Davis.

Pullen, R. L., Reed, K. E., & Oslar, K. S. (2001). Promoting clinical scholarship through scholarly writing. *Nurse Educator, 26*(1), 81–83.

Reed, P. G., & Zurakowski, T. L. (1996). Nightingale: Foundations of nursing. In J. J. Fitzpatrick & A. L. Whall (Eds.), *Conceptual models of nursing: Analysis and application* (3rd ed., pp. 55–76). Stamford, CT: Appleton & Lange.

Rogers, E. M. (2003). *Diffusion of innovation.* New York: Free Press.

Rosswurm, M. A., & Larrabee, J. H. (1999). A model for change to evidence-based practice. *Image: Journal of Nursing Scholarship, 31,* 317.

Sackett, D. L., Rosenberg, W. M., Gray, J. A., Haynes, R. B., & Richardson, W. S. (1996). Evidence based medicine: What it is and what it isn't. *British Medical Journal, 312*(7023), 71–72.

Schlotfeldt, R. M. (1992). Why promote clinical nursing scholarship? *Clinical Nursing Research, 1*(1), 5–8.

Sigma Theta Tau Clinical Scholarship Task Force. (1999a, November). *Clinical scholarship white paper.* Paper presented at the 35th Biennial Convention of Sigma Theta Tau International, San Diego, CA.

Sigma Theta Tau Clinical Scholarship Task Force. (1999b). *Clinical scholarship resource paper.* Retrieved December 4, 2010, from http://www.nursingsociety.org/aboutus/PositionPapers/Documents/clinical_scholarship_paper.pdf

Smith, M. J., & Liehr, P. R. (Eds.). (2003). *Middle range theory for nursing.* New York: Springer.

Stetler, C., Brunell, M., Biuliano, K., Morsi, D., Prince, L., & Newell-Stokes, G. (1998). Evidence-based practice and the role of nursing leadership. *Journal of Nursing Administration, 28*(7/8), 45–53.

Stillwell, S. B., Fineout-Overholt, E., Melnyk, B. M., & Williamson, K. M. (2010). Asking the clinical question: A key step in evidence-based practice. *American Journal of Nursing, 110*(3), 58–61.

Sussman, S., Valente, T. W., Rohrbach, L. A., Skara, S., & Pentz, M. A. (2006). Translation in the health professions. *Evaluation & the Health Professions, 29*(1), 7–32.

Thal, W. R. (2010). *Use of standards of care by nurse practitioners in providing care to adolescents with asthma at an academic nurse managed primary care clinic.* Unpublished manuscript, College of Nursing, The University of Arizona, Tucson.

University of Arizona College of Nursing. (2010). *Guidelines for preparation of the doctor of nursing practice.* Unpublished manuscript, College of Nursing, The University of Arizona, Tucson.

Wright, L. M., & Leahey, M. (2000). Nurses and families: A guide to family assessment and intervention (3rd ed.). Philadelphia: F. A. Davis.

INTERLUDE IV

Community-Based Nursing Praxis as a Catalyst for Generating Knowledge

Cathleen Michaels
Pamela G. Reed

*N*urses walk many paths in practice that can generate knowledge for the discipline. One path is community. As health care reform becomes reality, nurses increasingly will practice in community moving beyond the walls of hospitals, clinics, and office practices to enhance the health of individuals, families, and other groups in places where people live, work, play, and pray. This chapter focuses on community-based practice as a context for generating nursing knowledge. An overall goal is to provide real-life examples, drawn from Dr. Michael's community-based practice and research, of how action links to theory; that is, how community-based practices can be catalysts for developing theoretical ideas and concepts that can inform practice. A final goal is to increase nurses' awareness that theory—meaning ideas about relevant concepts and how they may be related to understand or explain a health-related process or concern—is embedded in community practice where people need coaching and guiding in everyday approaches to protecting health and managing chronic conditions.

Nursing practice in community either with individuals or groups can also be a catalyst for knowledge production by community members. Paulo Freire (1970), an internationally renowned educational progressive, advocated knowledge production by ordinary people for identifying and resolving problems in everyday life. In our case, nurses' and community members' knowledge production creates opportunity to integrate knowledge for the purpose of working together toward health-related goals. Community is a natural context where nurses and community members partner to foster health and health-related knowledge for human welfare.

PERSPECTIVES ON COMMUNITY

Community may be defined geographically or relationally. An example of a community defined geographically is the population of a city with defined boundaries.

An example of a community defined relationally is a group of people with chronic obstructive pulmonary disease (COPD) living in close proximity but not necessarily in the same town who meet monthly to discuss approaches to self-managing COPD. With either definition, the essential characteristic of community is a shared identity and interaction between community members (Israel, Checkoway, Schulz, & Zimmerman, 1994; Wilkinson, 1991).

Although the geographical definition prevails in health care, other perspectives about community are helpful for nurses to maintain while working with a community. These perspectives alert nurses to characteristics and resources within a community to draw from in facilitating community-based projects and interventions. In particular, McKnight (1992) provided a perspective about the potential of community, viewing community in terms of its members' strengths for working together to solve problems. McKnight (1992) drew from ideas by Alexis de Tocqueville, the French count who visited the United States in 1831 and observed something new among the American citizens:

> First, they were groups of citizens who decided they had the power to decide what was a problem. Second, they decided they had the power to decide how to solve the problem. Third, they often decided that they would themselves become the key actors in implementing the solution. (pp. 57–58)

A community can-do spirit reflects a readiness the nurse can build on in working toward health goals for individuals within a community or the community as a whole.

ASSESSING INFLUENCES ON COMMUNITY CAPACITY FOR HEALTH

As nurses, we are accustomed to describing health in terms of individuals, yet we are also aware that individuals are embedded in various systems or "influential spheres" (Labonte, 1993), including social, cultural, and physical environments. Labonte (1993) explained that if we overemphasize health at the individual level, our practice will define health as an individual process and disregard the significant influence of small groups (such as family and relational communities), geographic community, larger organizations, and the environment on health. He noted that the small group, such as the relational community, was particularly influential for the interpersonal bonds and social support it can provide.

Overall, without this larger perspective of influential spheres, for example, a nurse may offer a treatment plan to an individual newly diagnosed with diabetes but disregard how her family influences her eating habits or disregard the social and economic underpinnings that may limit accessibility to health care services and professional support. *Community capacity* for health, that is the human and material resources needed to make a desired change (Norton, McLeroy, Burdine, Felix, & Dorsey, 2002), is increased by these many spheres of community influence. Successful community-based practice is more likely, then, when the nurse understands the contribution of small and large groups to health and can assess and apply the resources of these spheres.

Power relationships also influence community capacity for health and the success of community-based practice. If power is not shared within the community, community capacity to recognize and respond to health issues decreases. The nurse therefore must foster mutuality with community members. Forces that counteract mutuality include ascribing power to the person with the most education and the most resources as well as holding differing agendas by the nurse, researchers, and communities. Mutuality between nurse and client is mirrored in elements like who has the power to name the problem, make decisions, and manage resources (Labonte, 1997). Power relationships can be overt and subtle or covert. For a successful community-based practice, it is essential to analyze and monitor power relationships to establish and sustain mutuality.

COMMUNITY PRAXIS: A PERSPECTIVE UNDERLYING COMMUNITY-BASED PRACTICE

Praxis is the action process through which knowledge can be generated in the context of community-based practice. While there are many perspectives on praxis presented in the literature, from Aristotle to present philosophers, praxis was a key concept for critical theory and social science that emphasized emancipating people to think independently (Carr & Kemmis, 1986). Newman (1994), among several nurse scholars, provides a useful perspective for nursing praxis, explaining praxis as the integration of theory, practice, and research that facilitates health as expanding consciousness.

Both professional and people's praxis organize knowledge into theoretical relationships, apply the theory, evaluate the application, and then evaluate the outcomes. As elaborated by Freire in his 1970 book *Cultural Action for Freedom* (cited in Carr & Kemmis, 1986), outcomes generated through praxis develop through a back and forth between thought and action without a predetermined endpoint. Newman's nursing praxis emphasizes a focus on patterns in the back and forth process between thought and action. In terms of community-based projects and interventions, both types of praxis occur in the community and can create shared knowledge with the nurse as the empirical expert about health, process, and pattern recognition, and the client as expert about the details that form the patterns and their associated meanings.

Nursing praxis begins with bringing a nursing theoretical perspective about human beings and health to bear on nursing interactions with individuals and communities in a way that helps people recognize their own health patterns, definitions, and desires for health. In a community-based project, nursing praxis becomes a shared or *community praxis* when community members use knowledge of their own health patterns along with other knowledge sources to participate in health-promoting practices. Evaluations of these practices or actions are used to reform or refine the theoretical perspectives that will inform subsequent action. Knowledge and actions are evaluated by action research methods and then reflected on in terms of two outcomes: (a) expanded awareness about one's health patterns and

(b) tangible results of the action on health or health practices. Both outcomes can be transformative in bringing about changes in perspectives and behaviors.

RESPECTFUL DIALOGUE

According to Freire (1970) and Newman (1994), the foundation for praxis is respectful dialogue in which no one person dominates but power is equally shared through respect for each individual. Without the authenticity and value for multiple perspectives that underlie respectful dialogue, mutuality cannot emerge. Uneven power relationships or lack of mutuality can limit coparticipation in identifying and naming a problem as well as deciding how to respond to the problem with available resources.

CONSCIENTIZATION

Conscientization is a term coined by Freire (1970) to describe awareness of a process of consciousness-raising that must precede action. According to Freire in his 1970 book *Cultural Action for Freedom* (as cited in Carr & Kemmis, 1986), conscientization refers to a "… deepening awareness both of the sociohistorical reality which shapes their [people's] lives and of their capacity to transform that reality" (p. 157). Conscientization is based on an approach to teaching that emphasizes questioning mainstream ideas, beliefs, and practices by understanding deeper meanings and root causes. Freire considered conscientization a necessary first step, essential for people to connect their experiences with their social context and confidently consider action for change. For example, in Freire's (1970) Brazilian community, he educated the people not only to read but also to become aware that the inability to read exacerbated oppression of the poor because literacy was required to vote in public elections.

Likewise, Newman (1994) described a process by which clients could consciously connect their experiences into a pattern of the whole. For example, Newman described a method in which the client tells his life story, describing what is most meaningful in life. The client's story revealed person–environment themes about his health patterns over time. It is not uncommon for clients to meaningfully interact with their environment to promote health, particularly when chronic illness is present. In community-based practice, then, the nurse values and facilitates community member awareness of patterns that express inherent abilities to take a desired action that influences their health and well-being.

PARTICIPATORY ACTION RESEARCH

Community-based practice requires the nurse and community members to work together in planning and implementing action to benefit the health of community members of the community as a whole. The degree of community participation influences the effectiveness of the intervention, including the relevance of the knowledge that informs the action and the potential for ownership in sustaining the effort. However, community-based practice results not only in effecting change to promote health but also in generating knowledge for practice because it entails methods of research as well as nursing practice. The community-based process that insures full participation and meaningful outcomes aligns with the tenets of participatory action research. *Participatory action research* refers to a philosophy and research methods that place high value on knowing through action-based experience coupled with research methods (Reason, 1994). The action-based approach is organized by a cycle of "planning, acting, observing, and reflecting" (Carr & Kemmis, 1986, p. 162).

EXAMPLE OF COMMUNITY-BASED PRACTICE WITH A GROUP: THE TUCSON HOLISTIC HEALING INITIATIVE FOR NURSES (THHIN)

My work with the THHIN is an example of community praxis. THHIN is a partnership between the The University of Arizona College of Nursing and 5 original hospital partners, now 10 partners. The purpose of the partnership is to promote the health and well-being of hospital staff nurses by exploring and using holistic modalities and integrated therapies in the work place. Examples of these modalities include deep breathing techniques, aromatherapy, and music therapy.

The group initially convened, discussed, and decided on its purpose, named itself, and planned four consultations for the first year of the project. The consultations focused on creating healing environments and adopting holistic modalities and integrated therapies for work-based self-care practices. Following each consultation, a planning group, consisting of several representatives from each hospital partner and two nurse faculties who served as facilitators, met to reflect on and discuss the highlights of each consultation to make the next consultation more effective. Although the group began more like a traditional committee, a relational community developed early in the process based on a common interest in THHIN and frequent interactions.

Knowledge produced through the relational community included approaches to building community capacity and *social capital*, that is, the interpersonal bonds between community members and bridges between hospitals. At the start of THHIN, community capacity was low; indicating a need for more interactions to build social capital (Kreuter & Lezin, 2002). Meeting every 2 weeks for a month and then monthly resulted in a rapid increase in social capital as well as an increase in community capacity as human and other resources were mobilized to showcase the consultations.

As the project progressed, community members provided feedback about the consultations, which then was translated into decisions to modify the consultations. For example, community members decided to transform end-of-consultation meetings with each consultant and their respective chief nursing officers to fewer meetings over breakfast to insure that all would be present. In doing so, community members created their own theory about the process needed to conclude each consultation. Although this change was specific to the THHIN process, a similar process could be considered in developing other community-based partnerships.

A STORY ABOUT THE EVOLUTION OF A NURSING THEORY OF PARTNERSHIP THROUGH COMMUNITY-BASED PRACTICE WITH INDIVIDUALS

My community-based practice provides rich data about partnering with individuals and groups to promote health. Reflections on these experiences along with knowledge about community and my praxis perspective help me generate theoretical concepts out of my practice.

My initial community-based work was with individual patients. As I spoke to hospitalized patients about being able to support them in the community, I felt uncertain about whether I would be welcomed into discharged patient homes. In general, people feel vulnerable and in need of help when hospitalized but not so when they are in community. Moreover, I realized that patient homes were not professional turf. Nevertheless, I suggested continuing my support beyond the hospital walls. I introduced myself and said that I would like to offer my support to help with any health concerns. In response, patients usually asked about what kind of help I meant. I then offered detailed examples based on the nature of their health. Then, one day, a hospital patient characterized my offer of help to her friend by explaining that the hospital had sent her a *partner*. In describing the process of this beginning relationship between nurse and patient then, I would say that a conversation had initiated relationship, the health issues and potential support established context for the relationship, and labeling the relationship as *partnership* moved the relationship beyond the hospital walls into the community.

During my visits in the community, I endeavored to deepen the relationships between myself and patients by, primarily, listening. I listened to patients tell stories about their illness experience, their sense of cause and consequence, and their perspectives about what makes them feel better and worse. My support of their understanding of illness and their acceptance of my questions and comments about their illness cocreated our relationship. In this relationship, we shared knowledge and acted together to better the patient's situation. As my relationship with a patient continued to unfold, the patient and I increased our sense of self and other—myself as person and nurse and the other as person and patient.

THEORETICAL CONCEPTS FROM PRACTICE

From reflections on my community-based practice with individual patients, I identified some key concepts and relationships, particularly as they illuminated *how* I engaged and sustained relationships with patients in the community. This interest in "how" and asking "how" questions underlies and generates theoretical thinking in and about practice.

The first concept to emerge in my theorizing was **connectedness**. I selected the concept of connectedness to refer to the *nature* of my relationships with patients, as they progressed from discussing hospital discharge to community. The initial connectedness varied and ranged from simply being invited into the patient's home to being welcomed with a thoughtfully planned tea party, as demonstrated by Helen, a 75-year-old patient and widow who lived alone in a senior community. My initial visit with Helen took place at her home since she had only been a patient in the emergency room, not the hospital. For my second home visit, Helen set up a tea table for two. She placed a white sheet over her coffee table and used her meager resources to provide tea and cake. Thus, I used connectedness to conceptually frame my work with patients in the community. By connectedness, I mean a genuine, authentic relationship between myself and the patient, which was mirrored by Helen's heartfelt actions in preparing the tea party for us to enjoy together.

The second concept I identified was **partnership** as inspired by a patient's characterization of my role with her in the community. I defined this concept as a *process*, referring to how the patient and I worked together as partners toward health-related goals. Our partnership was formed as we explicitly agreed to work together.

The third concept that I adopted was **mutual endeavor**. I described this concept in terms of the *content* of our relationship, which focused on our mutual goal of finding ways to enhance the patient's health situation. Without mutuality, a relationship is one sided and therefore not fully functional and unable to meet its potential.

The fourth concept I identified from my practice was **mutual benefit**. This concept reflects an *outcome* of the process of our partnership endeavor. Both the patient and I benefitted from the mutual endeavor, myself as a person and nurse and the patient as a person and patient. In most descriptions of nurse–patient relationship, the only benefits described are ascribed to the patient, as if the nurse did not experience personal and professional benefits. However, the nurse benefits as the dyadic relationship provides feedback to the nurse for professional as well as personal growth. Most notably, the nurse benefits from gaining professional knowledge that can be used to construct or build theory to guide other practice situations. Personally, the nurse benefits by having the opportunity to enact, question, evaluate, and modify values and beliefs about health through an encounter with another human being. Without acknowledging these positive experiences for the nurse, the nurse's authenticity cannot be fully established as true and genuine.

SCOTTY: AN EXAMPLE OF THE LINK BETWEEN ACTION AND THEORY

When I consider the theoretical concepts—particularly the concept of mutual benefit—that have emerged from my community-based practice, I think of my work with Scotty. Scotty was a 78-year-old community member and patient. He was an intriguing person—independent and living alone with no social support other than talking to the clerk in Walgreen's and who kept $10,000 in a jar in the refrigerator in case he "had to leave town quickly." Healthwise, he had a difficult time believing in physiology as dynamic and influenced by his health practices, as evidenced by his belief that a "good" blood pressure would be one where the systolic and diastolic values should always be the same number. Scotty confided that he was going to buy cedar berries and stop taking his oral antiglycemic agent. His evidence for making this decision was a physician letter to the editor in a local newspaper that declared diabetes can be cured with cedar berries.

While I had high personal value for Scotty's autonomy and self-determination, I also knew that unless he altered his health practices, Scotty could likely end up hospitalized again with hyperosmolar coma secondary to hyperglycemia. To acknowledge both of my perspectives, I affirmed to Scotty that it was his decision whether or not he took his medication or cedar berries, but I also suggested that he learn to monitor his blood glucose to know how his diabetes was responding. I was working from my belief in Scotty's inner strengths and from the idea that by helping Scotty learn more about his health patterns, he would make better informed decisions about his health practices related to his diabetes.

Scotty did learn to check his blood sugar using a glucometer. He became a reflective practitioner in a sense by systematically checking his blood sugar before and after meals and relating the results to different foods he ate and to his various activities such as walking around the block. After 3 months of measuring his blood sugar and recording the results, Scotty told me he decided to continue taking his diabetic medications because he did not want to "rock the boat." I breathed a sigh of relief because he had reflected and then chosen to continue this important self-management practice.

In reflecting on my own practice, I realized that my values for autonomy and self-determination coupled with my expert knowledge about diabetes and interpersonal relationships helped me create an effective glucose monitoring feedback system with Scotty. Through our partnership, which was buttressed by our connectedness, Scotty came to a better understanding of the influences and outcomes of glycemic control, which enabled and motivated him to decide to continue his medications. I approached our work as a mutual endeavor, accounting for both his values and mine in the interactions. The outcome was one of mutual benefit in that Scotty chose a health practice that would benefit him, and I gained knowledge for my work in the community. I also confirmed through another source that there is evidence that cedar berries lowers blood sugar. For me, this represented Scotty's own self-determination and wisdom that he brought to his own health care, which made us truly partners in his health care.

A COMMUNITY PRAXIS APPROACH TO PRACTICE AND KNOWLEDGE: A PERSONAL REFLECTION

The focus of the chapter has been on health-related action and knowledge production through partnership of the nurse and client (individual or community) in the community-based practice environment. As background, I discussed the importance of nurses understanding a community's inherent strengths and challenges, accounting for community identity and diversity, and assessing power relationships and other factors that influence community capacity for health. Examples of community-based practice were presented, along with my brief story of an evolving theory of partnership.

My practice with Scotty and Helen highlight my praxis perspective and partnership with patients. Professional and personal reflections on my practice in this and other encounters with individuals in the community have helped me develop theoretical ideas about the importance of nurse and patients joining together to form a partnership to improve the patient's health situation. So far, I have identified four concepts in my theory of community partnership, all positively related, so I may propose questions about the effects of connectedness, partnership, or mutuality on various health outcomes. In addition, as my community-based practice has come to include communities as clients, I have the opportunity to continue developing my theoretical ideas, for example, by examining how knowledge generated from practice with *individual* patients may inform action at the *community* level. A next step will be to organize these concepts into a theoretical framework that propose relationships between concepts to explain something unique about nurse–patient encounters in my community-based practice.

A central focus of the chapter was a discussion of *community praxis* as a perspective useful to nurses who engage a community in the coproduction of knowledge though community-based practice. The goals of community-based nursing practice are enhanced by engaging the community in praxis to address a given health concern by mutually deciding what the problem is, what to do about it, and how to know if the action is successful. Community praxis provides a perspective of partnering with individuals in the community, a partnership that helps support the inherent strengths of the members and community as a whole, while helping to free participants from social constraints and resolve problems to make a difference in their health and well-being. The perspective of community praxis coupled with skillful community-based interactions can foster a practice that builds both nursing knowledge and individual and community capacity to address problems in health-promoting ways.

QUESTIONS FOR REFLECTION

1. How would you evaluate the usefulness of the community praxis perspective presented here in your own work with patients?
2. How might you use the partnership approach to develop ideas for knowledge or theory development in your area of research?
3. What ideas do you have about other approaches to linking theory and practice that might extend or differ from the ideas presented in this chapter?
4. From your own experiences, what theoretical concepts might you identify that could be helpful in building theory to address the same health problem across different patients?

REFERENCES

Carr, W., & Kemmis, S. (1986). *Becoming critical: Education, knowledge and action research.* London: The Falmer Press.

Freire, P. (1970). *Pedagogy of the oppressed.* New York: The Seabury Press.

Israel, B. A., Checkoway, B., Schulz, A., & Zimmerman, M. (1994). Health education and community empowerment: Conceptualizing and measuring perceptions of individual, organizational, and community control. *Health Education Quarterly, 21,* 149–170.

Kreuter, M. W., & Lezin, N. (2002). Social capital theory: Implications for community-based health promotion. In R. J. DiClemente, R. A. Crosby, & M. C. Kegler (Eds.), *Emerging theories in health promotion, practice and research* (pp. 228–254). San Francisco, CA: Jossey-Bass.

Labonte, R. (1993). The empowerment holosphere. In R. Labonte (Ed.), *Health promotion and empowerment: Practice frameworks* (Issues in Health Promotion Series Monograph, HP-10–0102, pp. 59–89). Toronto, Ontario, Canada: Centre for Health Promotion, University of Toronto and ParticipACTION.

Labonte, R. (1997). Community, community development and the forming of authentic partnerships: Some critical reflections. In M. Minkler (Ed.), *Community organization and community building for health* (pp. 82–96). New Brunswick, NJ: Rutgers University Press.

McKnight, J. L. (1992). Redefining community. *Social Policy, 23*(2), 56–62.

Newman, M. (1994). *Health as expanding consciousness* (2nd ed.). New York, NY: National League for Nursing Press.

Norton, B. L., McLeroy, K. R., Burdine, J. N., Felix, M. R. J., & Dorsey, A. M. (2002). Community capacity. In R. J. DiClemente, R. A. Crosby, & M. C. Kegler (Eds.), *Emerging theories in health promotion, practice and research* (pp. 194–227). San Francisco, CA: Jossey-Bass.

Reason, P. (1994). Three approaches to participative inquiry. In N. K. Denzin & Y. S. Lincoln (Eds.), *Handbook of qualitative research* (pp. 324–339). Thousand Oaks, CA: Sage.

Wilkinson, K. (1991). *The community in rural America.* Westport, CN: Greenwood Press.

10

A Paradigm for the Production of Practice-Based Knowledge: Philosophical and Practical Considerations

Pamela G. Reed
Lisa A. Lawrence

No one owns science. If we wish to make informed choices, we must never forget that science exists because people created it, and it cannot exist separate from the community. Behind all the...professional degrees, the idea of science—our long effort to understand nature—and the knowledge that radiates from that search, are part of our shared human heritage.

   Ede & Cormack, 2004, p. 420

A PARADIGM FOR THE PRODUCTION OF PRACTICE-BASED KNOWLEDGE

From composers to scientists, innovation and discovery are highly valued by society and by the innovators themselves. Beethoven, for example, believed so deeply in innovation and individual expression above ritual and tradition that the originality of each of his nine symphonies limited him to composing far fewer symphonies than his predecessors (Grove, 1962). Conner's (2005) compelling account of the history of science reveals the significance of the artisans—people who worked with their hands—in the development of knowledge and the Scientific Revolution. The artisans transformed know-how into knowledge through the daily practices of their work, which involved ongoing experimentation, intervention, and the use of instruments. The birth of modern science occurred, Conner (2005) explains, when the intellectual elite engaged in "knowledge robbery," appropriating artisans' knowledge and then systematizing it. The artisans' "latent contribution to science" did not reap recognition as learned individuals, but it significantly advanced knowledge during the Middle Ages. Artisans' work also brought forth a method of knowledge production that connected the scientist to nature rather than ancient authority.

The contributions of caregiving nurses to the well-being of patients and the viability of health care systems are indisputable. Like the artisans of the past, caregiving nurses today are not recognized for their production of knowledge. In fact, within our current paradigm of knowledge development, most nurses are socialized into being users, not producers, of knowledge. This perspective is reinforced in nursing education as well as in practice. This chapter explores trends and issues surrounding knowledge production and nursing practice and proposes a paradigm of knowledge development that promotes nursing knowledge production among practicing nurses. *Nursing knowledge* refers to knowledge warranted as useful and significant to nurses and patients in understanding and facilitating human health processes.

THE KNOWLEDGE DISTINCTION IN A PROFESSION

One important characteristic of a profession is that its practice is accompanied by a dynamic system of knowledge development. The persons who develop knowledge are most frequently called scientists, scholars, and researchers, generally not practitioners. Nursing distinguishes between the knowledge producers and the knowledge users; those designated as the knowledge producers typically are educated in research doctoral programs rather than in practice-based undergraduate and graduate programs. This knowledge distinction within a discipline perpetuates ambiguity in professional standing and vulnerability to decreased jurisdiction over practice.

MARGINALIZING NURSING KNOWLEDGE

No professional nursing achievement is as paradoxical as the establishment of the National Institute for Nursing in the United States, "which recognizes and supports the professional status of nursing" while the occupational settings in which nursing is applied do not necessarily support educational preparation to enable all nurses to be knowledge producers (Lynaugh & Fagin, 2000, p. 48). For all they do and know, practitioners remain an untapped dimension of knowledge development in our discipline.

The American Association of Colleges of Nursing (2004) has identified those with research doctorates to be the knowledge producers of the discipline, who then transmit knowledge to nurses prepared at all other levels—baccalaureate, masters, and practice doctorate; this latter group of nurses are expected to "use and evaluate, but not conduct, research" (American Association of Colleges of Nursing, 2004, 2007). However, nursing is in need of more nurses who can expand, not just evaluate, its knowledge base. In addition, more nurses than those who possess the research doctoral degree may be capable of, and interested in, knowledge production. In the words of the French philosopher Michael Serres (1995), "it is better to do than to judge, to produce than to evaluate, to create than to criticize, to invent than to classify copies. Playing is better than blowing the referee's whistle" (p. 128). There is something unseemly in the suggestion that practitioners do evaluation research for their scholarship because they are "hampered by heavy practice or teaching workloads" (Eddy, 2007); practitioners, like knowledge developers, are confronted with new situations every time a patient walks through the door and are capable of integrating new information to explain how these situations are best dealt with (Lum, 2002).

Segregating knowledge users and evaluators from knowledge producers promotes an exclusive approach to knowledge generation where the few generate knowledge for the many. Current statistics indicate that less than 1% of nurses are developing knowledge for the other 99% of nurses: The most recent U.S. National Sample Survey of Registered Nurses (NSSRN) indicates the following distribution of educational degrees among the nearly 3 million registered nurses (RNs) in the United States: Doctoral in nursing or related field, 0.9%; Masters, 12%; Bachelor, 32%; Associate, 34%; Diploma, 17.5%; with the remaining unknown (U.S. Department of Health and Human Resources & Health Resources and Services Administration, 2007). Subdividing the 0.9% of doctoral-level nurses into those who are and who are not prepared to conduct independent research (that is, the research doctorate and practice doctorate, respectively) further hinders nursing's knowledge-production capacity. This segregation harkens memories of the media and the public questioning the nurse's right to engage in independent research and publication "without the imprimatur of a physician" (Downs, 1991, p. 195). Epistemological decisions about who are the legitimate knowers and knowledge producers in nursing have sociopolitical implications for practice (Bart, 2000). Clinicians who are perceived as lacking the ability to produce knowledge for their practice are more vulnerable to falling under the jurisdiction of other health care professionals.

Too many nurses still work from an impoverished knowledge base, in part because the discipline has not shaken loose an operative ontology of "physician's orders." Tens of thousands of nurses still follow physicians' orders and, in 17 states in the United States, they follow physician assistants' orders. It is inconsistent with professional practice that nursing practices are dependent on physicians' orders to implement nursing care, such as ambulating or turning patients, entering consults to other disciplines, and providing an on-the-spot normal saline spray for a person suffering from a bleeding nose as a result of exposure to dry, desert air. Rather than implementing practices consistent with the scope and focus of nursing knowledge, nurses spend exorbitant amounts of time preparing and passing medications that nurses do not prescribe and in implementing and coordinating medical treatments that nurses do not order.

Sociologist Andrew Abbott (1988) studied the system of professions and determined that abstract knowledge is a major element in a profession's level of jurisdiction or control over practice. He explained that professions have varying forms of jurisdiction over their practice: Some professions share jurisdiction over practice with each other, as with attorneys and certified public accountants; some have an advisory relationship, such as that between clergy and medicine; other professions have control over cognitive knowledge but not over their practice such as that between psychotherapists and psychiatrists. Abbott (1988) used nursing as the exemplar of the most limited form of jurisdiction over one's practice, which he called "subordination."

Abbott (1988) explained that a profession's jurisdiction over practice depends in large part on the educational level of the profession. However, perhaps more importantly, he found that level of jurisdiction was related to the presence of abstract thinking or theories used in practice. Mechanics, for example, are not professionals *per se*, but if they possessed the abstract knowledge of an engineer to link their observations and technical prowess to theoretical explanations, they could be. The same goes for caregivers and nursing knowledge. Jurisdiction and autonomy are difficult to achieve without the requisite knowledge and knowledge-building skills, no matter how gilded is the path from novice to expert.

BLACK-BOXING CAREGIVER KNOWLEDGE

The discipline of nursing grew out of a public demand for knowledgeable caregivers (Fagin, 2000), and nursing is recognized as the profession of caregiving. However, nurses' caregiving knowledge has been "black-boxed"—a metaphor used by Latour (1999) to indicate that a work or a technology "has been made invisible by its own success" (p. 304). Black-boxing occurs when a complexity of elements act as one. It is a metaphor symbolizing the closing off of continued interest, appreciation, and inquiry into a dynamic source of scientific knowledge and rendering it as an "opaque object of fact" (Sturman, 2006, p. 182).

Black-boxing occurs in nursing when the complexity of behaviors and ideas that come together in nurses' acts of caregiving are invisible and not well understood or fully appreciated; however, paradoxically, black-boxed knowledge is considered credible and too costly to understand or replace. Caregiving becomes transparent, a taken-for-granted yet integral reality of health care. Furthermore, what is "black-boxed" is considered compact and portable. The professional practice of cross-coverage and use of traveling nurses are visible examples of black-boxing nurses' caregiving knowledge and skills within nursing practice. Nurses are imported to practice within the context of a new unit. In so doing, knowledge is separated from the context of its discovery (Latour & Woolgar, 1986).

Without the active support of clinical leaders and managers, the inventiveness and originality inherent in nurses' daily caregiving work withers. We claim that to the extent that nursing and other health care professions do not recognize the knowledge potential and knowledge produced in the context of caregiving, but benefit from it, "knowledge robbery" occurs—similar to that which occurred among 16th-century artisans. This fuzzy focus on nursing caregiving behaviors can also discourage nurses' efforts to be innovative or pursue evidence and knowledge. Nurses may legitimize their practices only by moral or technical approaches to health care rather than by a scientific understanding of the full complexity of the human health problem and empowering patients in their health care (Nelson & Gordon, 2006).

EXTANT PARADIGMS OF PRACTICE KNOWLEDGE

Frustrations over the status of nursing—perceived instead as a technical trade or as a semiprofession—span the 20th and 21st centuries (Anderson, 2001; Segal, 1985). This deficit in nursing knowledge and nursing-ordered practices has created a vacuum, which two paradigms of practice knowledge, "evidence-based" and "expert intuitive-practitioner" (Purkis & Bjornsdottir, 2006), have rushed in to fill. Each paradigm offers important perspectives for nursing practice but is insufficient for supporting nurse clinicians as knowledge-workers.

Evidence-based practice is usually broad enough to include the clinician's judgment and patient preferences and values, along with empirical evidence on clinical effectiveness of a treatment. However, it emphasizes knowledge packaged ahead of time for use, irrespective of the particular context and current contingencies. Evidence-based practice seeks to access knowledge, not to develop knowledge; it does not seek to answer questions about what is actually wrong with a patient and about the underlying mechanisms of the patient's problem and potential solutions (Fineout-Overholt, Melnyk, & Schultz, 2005; Roberts & Yeager, 2004). To be an empowered professional with jurisdiction over practice, nurses need to be able to participate in knowledge production.

The *intuitive-expert paradigm* of nursing practice originated with the work of Benner's (1984) *From Novice to Expert* and depicts the nurse as an "intuitive knower" and "primary judge" of the legitimacy of the nurse's clinical knowledge (Purkis & Bjornsdottir, 2006, p. 250). This model is practitioner-centered with a focus on the present context. It lacks the advantage of an external perspective and critique to inform nurses' judgments about what is "emancipating, good, healthful, and other value-laden concepts" that influence nursing judgment (Reed, 2006a). In addition, experience and expert-based sources of knowledge such as craft knowledge, know-how, or tacit knowledge represent the mystery and complexity of how professional practitioners think (Montgomery, 2006); however, equating these types of knowledge with nurses' practice knowledge and then rendering them ineffable stifles nursing's ability both to develop knowledge in and for practice, and to marshal evidence of the effectiveness of nursing knowledge, judgment, and skill.

Related to this intuitive-expert model is what Nelson and Gordon (2006) describe as a "narrowed caring discourse," which minimizes recognition of the technical, scientific, and physical practices involved in providing health care and contributes to a simplistic view of nursing care and nursing knowledge by the public and politicians. This "new Cartesianism" focuses on the interpersonal relationship and emotional connection while ignoring the "skills and complexity of body work" (p. 4). They criticize nurses and nursing organizations' heavy emphasis on nurses' virtues rather than on observable, knowledge-based contributions; this "virtue script" is impossible to enact satisfactorily in a hierarchical health care system where it instead "trivializes" nurses' complexity and competencies (Nelson & Gordon, 2006).

In addition to these practice knowledge models, research utilization, knowledge application, and translational research may also be viewed as strategies to fill gaps of scientific knowledge in practice. The effectiveness of these efforts along with those associated with evidence-based practice and caring-focused practice could be bolstered by a paradigm of practice-based knowledge production that recognizes, facilitates, and promotes practicing nurses as knowledge producers.

A PARADIGM OF PRACTICE-BASED KNOWLEDGE

Philosophers and scientists are embracing a pluralistic view of science and knowledge development that will facilitate greater participation of nurses, and all professionals, in knowledge development. This pluralistic view is found in the following contemporary philosophies: Carper's (1978) multiple patterns of knowing; Da Costa and French's (2003) idea of partial truths; Longino's (2002) philosophy of critical contextual empiricism; and Reed's (1995, 2006b) neomodernist view of knowledge. Gibbons et al. (1994) described the now widely referenced approach called *Mode 2 Knowledge Production* (also see Delanty, 2001). In this mode, knowledge production is characterized by its heterogeneity (bringing together diverse skills and experiences to address a problem); reflexivity (involving reflection on values and perspectives of all actors involved); and transdisciplinarity (where knowledge is context sensitive and problem oriented and may transcend traditional disciplinary boundaries, such as those between the university and health care center). Andrew Pickering (1995) captured some of this new view of knowledge production in a way quite applicable to clinical practice with his description of science as a "mangle" of social, technical, conceptual, political, and personal practices.

This expanded view of knowledge paves the way for knowledge production in clinical practice settings and provides for a more distinct role for practice knowledge—for example, as a "science of the unique" (Rolfe, 2006) in knowledge development. Practice itself is viewed as a generative source, if not a prerequisite, to developing nursing knowledge and theory (Reed, 1995). A pluralistic view of nursing knowledge still values the empirical and the theoretical, and the traditional role of critique and consensus in establishing truths; but what qualifies as empirical has gone beyond empiricism to include qualitative as well as quantitative data, stories, and words as well as measures and numbers. This view also takes into account the influences on knowledge development of such social factors of science as the method and context of inquiry (clinical or laboratory, for example), values and beliefs of the knowledge producer, and the relationship of the researcher to the researched.

Conceptual, practical, and technological innovations are all valued for their role in helping nurses provide better patient care. The potential benefits of knowledge production and innovation by nurses are phenomenal, irrespective of the form of innovation, as indicated in the following examples: Discovering how to use the theoretical concept of "expanding consciousness" to facilitate patient well-being at the end of life (Barron, 2005) and "pattern recognition" to enhance the well-being of women with multiple sclerosis (Neill, 2005); developing a new professional development model that reduces cost and increases nurses' work effectiveness and satisfaction (Bournes & Ferguson-Paré, 2007); adapting an existing evidence-based oral care program for the needs of a specific nursing unit to decrease non-ventilator-associated pneumonia (Federwisch, 2007); or innovating a nursing procedure that hastens healing of a below-the-knee amputation (Dolde, 2007).

The purpose in pluralism is not to remedy inadequacies in any one method of knowledge production alone through some relativist view or to synthesize or resolve paradoxes but to construct places that can sustain the conversation to explore and develop a variety of approaches for their value in building knowledge and solving problems. "Paradoxical, creative thinking, tempered by tolerance for ambiguity is essential in nursing science practice and it…distinguishes the clinical expert in nursing science from the rigid and rule-bound procedural technician in nursing" (Rawnsley, 2000, p. 232).

THEORY: A TOOL OF KNOWLEDGE DEVELOPMENT

The 21st-century and post-postmodern perspectives (Reed, 1995) have ushered in new thinking about nursing theory consistent with the paradigm of practice-based knowledge presented above. Theory as redefined within these new perspectives is a useful tool for practitioners in knowledge development and in achieving the level of abstract knowledge needed to support jurisdiction over practice (Abbott, 1988). Rigid application and preservation of nursing theories understandably have chilled nurses' appreciation for theories' roles in practice. It is not so much that theories are too abstract or difficult to understand as much as they constrain nursing practice and creativity when regarded as an unchangeable voice of authority.

Within this new paradigm of knowledge production, theories are not meant to be applied in a cook-book manner directly to practice but rather to be used, modified, and indeed developed in conjunction with the nurse's creative critical reasoning and interactions with patients. In this way, theory can accommodate the "unforeseeable moments" and reflect an understanding of the way "nursing is lived in practice" (Salas, 2005, p. 22).

The word *theory* is used here to refer to conceptualizations at all levels of abstraction, from broad conceptual frameworks to theories focused on a specific situation (Higgins & Moore, 2000). A theory defined broadly is a dynamic system of concepts that provides an organized perspective, explanation, or probabilistic prediction of an aspect of reality or human experience. This system of concepts also connects us with a larger perspective of the world that cannot be seen from within the immediate context of discovery. Theories are the building blocks of knowledge in a discipline. They provide a degree of effectiveness, dependability, and longevity useful in practice, although every theory is tentative. Theories can move the practitioner beyond the present to facilitate some understanding of "principles, processes and mechanisms that produce or underlie what is present to us" (Longino, 2002, p. 124). In addition, theories may be transported to other relevant contexts for use, beyond the one where they were generated.

Within a pluralistic view of knowledge development, truth is relational, not representational; theories derive their meaning through participation of all of those who share certain practices within a nursing community rather than from correspondence to some fixed indicator of reality (Reed, 2001). Scientific theory does not have to be universal or meet the claim that it will always apply, but it has to stand up to criteria and criticism by a relevant community, such as a certain community of patients or caregivers. Longino (2002) explains that this criticism involves showing how the theory's claims have been systematically generated, how they meet certain goals of the community, and then being open to making needed modifications. For example, modifications may be needed in the scope of the theory's claims or in the knowledge production or research process itself.

The nature of nursing—involving daily encounters with the complexity, uniqueness, and the unpredictability of human beings' health needs—requires that nurses think theoretically and speak of their knowledge. Nurses look for patterns, make connections, posit possible explanations about their observations, and test out and revise their ideas as the situation changes. Nurses are encouraged to question prevailing paradigms of knowledge development that may inhibit their own creative thinking (Meleis & Im, 1999).

The use of theory-based knowledge distinguishes the technical from the professional. Technical workers use what is at hand with less thought about reflecting on their own theories or importing other ideas to explain why things work. This at-handness is the realm of the practical, the immediate, and the unmediated. However, professional workers, members of a discipline, import materials, theories, skills, and technology from elsewhere to enhance their work (Ingraham, 1998).

KNOWLEDGE PRODUCTION IN PRACTICE: STRATEGIES AND INNOVATIONS

Professional practice is a theory-based service to society. Conceptualizing knowledge development as part of practice helps to sustain a dynamic knowledge system. While physicians bemoan the nurse staffing shortage because of their own "overwork and frustration" (Mangan, 2007), the crisis may also be viewed as a shortage of nursing practice *knowledge* that deprives patients from the full benefits of nursing. The need for nursing knowledge is great, given the increasing complexity of health care. New thinking that integrates practice and knowledge production opens up opportunities for caregiving nurses, with support from nurse managers, to participate more actively in knowledge development. Exactly how practitioners integrate abstract knowledge into the helping process is a scholarly area of study itself across disciplines in terms of how theory is linked with practice (e.g., Bug, 2000; Purkis & Bjornsdottir, 2006; Rolfe, 1998; Trierweiler & Stricker, 1998; Tucker, Garvin, & Sarri, 1997). For now, we offer a few strategies for nurses and nurse managers to consider, aware that each work environment presents unique challenges and opportunities for practice-based knowledge production.

PROMOTING THEORETICAL THINKING

The mindful use of theory separates the technical from the professional worker. In addition, the verbalization and continual development of theory is an essential component for professional advancement and the delivery of high-quality nursing care. Practitioners already possess cognitive and experiential skills to engage in theoretical thinking (Marrs & Lowry, 2006). The clinician is well placed to investigate the patient's problem and context and determine whether the patient's healing process can be accounted for by current theory and evidence or if some modification or an entirely new theory is needed instead.

Specific strategies are available that can be used to support practitioners' efforts in building knowledge. Forums, seminars, journal clubs, and other periodic meetings provide opportunities for nurses to meet (online or face to face) to discuss the latest thinking on a problem and reflect on practice. Topics may range from specific concrete problems in practice to reflection on personal philosophies about nursing, truth, life and death, and health and well-being. Knowledge production inevitably involves philosophical and ethical questions.

Ratner (2007) recently reported on an innovative strategy initiated by Marie Manthy, a nurse and president emeritus of Creative Healthcare Management, called a *nursing salon*, where nurses from diverse backgrounds meet monthly in a private home to discuss nursing-related issues. A facilitator maintains the focus on the selected theme. Manthy borrowed this concept from the historical practice of assembling notable artists, politicians, and writers in a private home for lively discussion and debate.

Reflection in practice has been identified as a particularly effective strategy for producing knowledge in practice and generating nursing theory (e.g., Johns, 2004; Palmer, Burns, & Bulman, 1994; Rolfe, 1998). Since Schön's (1983) seminal work on the reflective practitioner in education, scholars have acquired evidence of the significance of this approach in theoretical thinking among nursing practitioners (Clark, James, & Kelly, 1996; Peden-McAlpine, Tomlinson, Forneris, Genck, & Meiers, 2005).

Similar approaches for generating theory and knowledge that beg for more study and systematic use by practitioners are Pesut and Herman's (1999) outcome-present-state-test (OPT) model of reflective clinical reasoning and Peirce, Harshorne, and Weiss's (1934) abductive reasoning. These forms of reasoning are especially critical in our climate of evidence-based practice. It is not enough to know that an intervention works; it is important to know why and how it works (Lum, 2002). Theoretical thinking provides the means to better understand and judge the evidence for the well-being of individual patients. The resources for promoting theoretical thinking in practice are abundant.

PROMOTING USE OF CLINICAL CONCEPTUAL FRAMEWORKS

A mechanism for enhancing dialogue for knowledge production in practice is what we are calling the *clinical conceptual framework*, a more abstract kind of theory that is especially useful in practice-based knowledge production. Promoting knowledge development among practicing nurses depends on their ability to clearly articulate their operative frameworks and to develop their personal theories (Rolfe, 1998; Trierweiler & Stricker, 1998). Conceptual frameworks are an effective first step in theorizing—that is, in transforming observations, interactions, and other data into a form of theory—because it is easier to work with broader, less detailed concepts when beginning to organize ideas about some phenomenon. Conceptual frameworks are less specific than theories; they simplify structures, highlight the phenomena of interest, and provide a transportable model of some aspect of interest to the practitioner as knowledge producer (Lenoir, 1997). Conceptual frameworks facilitate knowledge production by mapping out the general territory of inquiry, suggesting questions to be asked and observations to be made.

Clinical conceptual frameworks may resemble extant nursing theories or they may be unique to the practitioner and the concepts she or he finds relevant in practice. Frameworks are flexible conceptual innovations. They may point to general laws of human functioning, or they may portray a process of change or well-being that is relevant to the practice situation at hand. Reflective practice cannot work unless guided by a framework that has been made explicit to the practitioner and others (Schön, 1983). Toward this end, nurse managers could encourage presentation and discussion of clinical conceptual frameworks on a regularly scheduled basis, such as quarterly.

Nurses may use conceptual frameworks to build knowledge with other professionals or with patients, for example, by unmasking misconceptions, positing radically different perspectives of health processes, and helping patients to clarify their experiences and illuminate new meanings of health (Seigfried, 1996). Philosophers of science suggest that conceptual models or frameworks facilitate dialogue between research and theory because models are at the same time models of observed phenomena and models of theory (Lenoir, 1997).

The practitioner can extend knowledge beyond that found in close readings of the canon (the extant conceptual frameworks) and inspire development of bold, new frameworks for deriving hypotheses and practice innovations. In a closed system of knowledge development dominated by traditional scientist views about reality, which assumes that there is a fixed theory or reality independent of mind and language, scientific progress would end once all that there is to discover is discovered (Horgan, 1996). However, the clinical conceptual framework, as part of a dynamic knowledge system, is a mechanism for handling new sources of knowledge brought in through the practitioner's daily interfaces with society. These interfaces create possibilities for new knowledge to emerge that cannot be explained by existing laws. Carrier (2000) called this a process of emergence, where new ideas cannot be explained by existing knowledge. *Caregiving is a gateway to emergent theories for nursing practices.*

PROMOTING PARTNERSHIPS FOR KNOWLEDGE PRODUCTION

Knowledge sharing between clinicians and academics occurs more readily when knowledge is regarded as a gift rather than a commodity, that is, as something to be shared and refined among people committed to understanding and promoting health. Thatchenkery and Chowdhry (2007) describe a process of knowledge management called *appreciative inquiry* that facilitates knowledge generation by accessing knowledge from outside sources. They labeled the specific strategy *appreciative sharing of knowledge* (ASK) that is used to generate and transfer knowledge across systems or organizations. Considering that clinical and academic institutions each have resources the other can use in knowledge production, we suggest that each institution use the strategies of ASK to share resources. For example, clinical scholars would benefit from having access to academic-type resources associated with library searches, statistical analyses, and preparing publications. Knowledge production entails thinking, reading, and technology.

Another suggestion is that clinical settings sanction some time and space for nurses (clinicians and academics) to exchange theoretical ideas as part of their professional responsibilities. As a recent example, the Veterans' Affairs Health Care System formalized a clinical and academic affiliation via the development of a VA Nursing Academy, a 5-year pilot project initiated to enhance partnerships between practice and academia (Department of Veterans Affairs, Veterans Health Administration, 2007). The VA Nursing Academy represents a mutually beneficial relationship between nursing schools and VA facilities; it is a partnership that encourages increases in student enrollments, especially at the baccalaureate level (p. 3) and promotes interprofessional learning and the scholarly development of projects related to the care of veterans.

As universities become more like firms and firms or hospitals become more like universities (Delanty, 2001), institutions may swap strategies to promote knowledge production. For example, hospitals could mandate hours (that are figured into staffing ratios) dedicated to education, sabbaticals, and participation in research conferences for practitioners. Bournes and Ferguson-Paré (2007) described an innovation by which nurses spent 80% of their salaried time in direct patient care and 20% time on professional development. Positive outcomes included increased patient and staff satisfaction and nonexistent turnover.

PROMOTING ATTAINMENT OF BACCALAUREATE-AND-HIGHER DEGREES

Nurses at all three professional educational levels are capable of engaging in abstract, reflective thinking in practice and are a resource for nursing knowledge production.

The link between baccalaureate-and-higher degree attainment and patient outcomes and mortality has been widely publicized (AACN website; Aiken, Clark, Cheung, Slone, & Silber, 2003; Long, 2004). Higher education enhances nurses' abilities to both use and develop new knowledge for practice. One of the most substantial changes in the RN population over the past quarter century has been their educational preparation. According to the most recent NSSRN (U.S. Department of Health and Human Resources & Health Resources and Services Administration, 2007) of 3 million RNs, the percentage of nurses who have obtained baccalaureate and higher degrees is on the rise. Between 1980 and 2004, the percentage of nurses enrolled in baccalaureate programs increased by 170%, those with master's or doctorate-level education quadrupled with a 339% increase, and there was an unprecedented 37% increase in the number of master's and doctorally prepared nurses. Diploma-level nurses decreased by 44% and continue to decline each year. These trends are promising in terms of the increasing number of professional nurses for practice and knowledge production.

Within the past few years, the American Association of Colleges of Nursing (AACN, 2004, 2007) has worked to establish two new degree programs in the United States: The Clinical Nurse Leader (CNL), a master's-level generalist degree with management and direct care focuses, and the Doctor of Nursing Practice (DNP), a practice doctorate and terminal degree for nurses. Both programs will accelerate the numbers of practicing nurses who can function as knowledge producers.

Specific strategies to promote nurses' attainment of higher degrees include clinical–university partnerships for financial support of students; creative and flexible work scheduling; providing clinical resources for coursework and educational study; and offering ongoing moral support and encouragement. A long-term strategy to coordinate with clinical leaders is twofold: (a) consolidate baccalaureate and master's nursing practice education programs to focus resources on educating more graduate degree nurses as clinical scholars; these clinical scholars would be leaders in applying and generating nursing theory and knowledge in their practice; and (b) maintaining the education of associate degree nurses who enact nursing practices and contribute to nursing knowledge under the nursing orders and guidance of clinical scholars.

THE PRACTITIONER AS CLINICAL SCHOLAR

It is also important for managers and educators to appreciate practitioners as clinical scholars. They participate in both the application of knowledge through practice and in the production of knowledge through inquiry. In addition, the clinical scholar is able to partner with researchers and patients in developing practice-based knowledge. Clinical scholars are skilled at interfacing with various contexts to develop knowledge. They are pivotal in bringing together the objective perspectives of the researcher and scientist, the subjective views of the patient, and their own patterns of knowing—personal, empirical, ethical, aesthetic, sociopolitical.

Clinical scholars are knowledge managers, sifting, analyzing, and discerning what is important in a diversity of data. However, the data will not yield up theories by themselves. So, clinical scholars are also knowledge producers—linking empirical to the theoretical to explain events and helping patients recognize patterns and meaning in what they are experiencing so they can participate more fully in their own health. The clinical scholar regards knowledge as process, not product. The answers are never final because patient contexts and conditions change, and knowledge itself changes. Clinical scholars use theories to help them anticipate change and see the bigger picture.

Clinical scholars are also leaders. They inspire and guide other nurses through knowledge-based practice. In addition, they reclaim the associate degree nurse from medicine. Associate degree nurses are the predominant nursing group in practice. Data from the 2004 NSSRN indicate that between 1980 and 2004, nurses enrolled in associate degree programs increased by 232%, where enrollments in baccalaureate programs increased by 170%. Although these enrollments leveled out between 2000 and 2004 at 13% for both programs, the highest educational degree for employed RNs is the associate degree at 34%, followed by the baccalaureate degree at 32%. Approaches to knowledge production that embrace associate degree nurses will be more successful than those that marginalize this group. Associate degree nurses can provide added workforce in nursing knowledge development as well as patient care under the supervision and orders of clinical scholars. By virtue of their large numbers, associate degree nurses can enhance nursing jurisdiction over practice by taking their orders from *nurses*. Clinical scholars would provide the supervision and nursing orders for associate degree nurses who remain the predominant nursing group in practice.

LOOKING FORWARD: THE *EDGE EFFECT*

The new wave of thinking about knowledge production recognizes the synergy in bringing together two systems: the system of knowledge development and the system of practice. This is evident by the prevalence of terms such as clinical scholar, practitioner/researcher, scholarly practitioner, and scientist-clinician in the literature and in our conversations. Where practice and research meet creates an *edge effect*, a term used to describe what happens when two ecosystems come together. The renowned cellist Yo-Yo Ma used this term to explain the productive interactions of culturally diverse edges of his life and art (Keller, 2007). The edge effect has the "least density and the greatest variety" (Keller, 2007) and generates new ideas and innovations. Similarly, philosopher Michael Serres (1995) described the interface between systems, such as between science and art, as "the place where things happen." With help from clinical leaders and managers, the practice setting can be a place where innovation and the development of new knowledge can happen.

Having a voice in the underlying ideas and direction of one's practice can be a pivotal element in promoting quality nursing care and in attracting and retaining nurses in the profession. We agree with Anderson (2001), in her commentary on how to achieve a culture of excellence and achievement amid the "challenged" status of nursing: "To surpass the current level...stretch the boundary of what is possible, be intolerant of the ordinary, be creative ..." (p. 209). May this paradigm of practice-based knowledge production become a movement away from the traditional, normal science and into what Kuhn (1962/1996) called "extraordinary science"—a period of ferment and theoretical experimentation in which the practices and concepts of so-called normal science are loosened in ever more radical ways in response to a persistent problem that resists solution within the limits of the prevailing normal science paradigm.

QUESTIONS FOR REFLECTION

1. What do you perceive are some potential benefits of practice-based knowledge production in advancing patient care?
2. What are potential challenges of practice-based knowledge production given the current climate in health care? What are some ways to meet these challenges for the benefit of nursing and patient care?
3. What ideas do you have about potential innovations or strategies in health care settings (your own or in general) that would support your activities as a knowledge-producer in practice?
4. What strategies mentioned in this chapter appeal to you in your role as a knowledge-producer in nursing? (e.g., promoting partnerships, developing a clinical conceptual framework, or what?)
5. Do you think that practice-based knowledge development is important in advancing the voice of nursing in health care?

REFERENCES

Abbott, A. (1988). *The system of professions*. Chicago: University of Chicago Press.

Aiken, L. H., Clark, S. P., Cheung, R. B., Slone, D. M., & Silber, J. H. (2003). Educational levels of hospital nurses and surgical patient mortality. *Journal of the American Medical Association, 290*, 1617–1623.

American Association of Colleges of Nursing. (2004). *Position Statement on the practice doctorate in nursing*. Washington, DC: Author.

American Association of Colleges of Nursing. (2007). *White paper on the education and role of the clinical nurse Leader*. Retrieved December 6, 2010, from http://www.aacn.nche.edu/Publications/WhitePapers/ClinicalNurseLeader.htm

Anderson, C. A. (2001). A culture of excellence and achievement. *Nursing Outlook, 49*, 209.

Barron, A. (2005). Suffering, growth and possibility: Health as expanding consciousness in end-of-life care. In C. Picard & D. Jones (Eds.), *Giving voice to what we know* (pp. 43–52). Boston: Jones and Bartlett.

Bart, J. (2000). Feminist theories of knowledge. In J. Bart (Ed.), *Women succeeding in the sciences: Theories and practices across disciplines* (pp. 205–220). West Lafayette, IN: Purdue University Press.

Benner, P. (1984). *From novice to expert.* Menlo Park, CA: Addison-Wesley.

Bournes, D. A., & Ferguson-Paré, M. (2007). Human becoming and 80/20: An innovative professional development model for nurses. *Nursing Science Quarterly, 20,* 237–253.

Bug, A. (2000). Gender and physical science: A hard look at a hard science. In J. Bart (Ed.), *Women succeeding in the sciences: Theories and practices across disciplines* (pp. 221–244). West Lafayette, IN: Purdue University Press.

Carper, B. A. (1978). Fundamental patterns of knowing in nursing. *Advances in Nursing Science, 1*(1), 13–23.

Carrier, M. (2000). *Science at century's end: Philosophical questions on the progress and limits of science.* Pittsburgh, PA: University of Pittsburgh Press.

Clark, B., James, C., & Kelly, J. (1996). Reflective practice: Reviewing the issues and refocusing the debate. *International Journal of Nursing Studies, 33,* 171–180.

Conner, C. D. (2005). *A people's history of science: Miners, midwives, and "low mechanics."* New York: Nation.

Da Costa, N. C. A., & French, S. (2003). *Science and partial truth: A unitary approach to models and scientific reasoning.* New York: Oxford University Press.

Delanty, G. (2001). *Challenging knowledge: The university in the knowledge society.* Philadelphia: Open University Press.

Department of Veterans Affairs, Veterans Health Administration. (2007). *VA nursing academy: Enhancing academic partnerships, starting in academic year 2007–2008, Request for Proposals.* Retrieved December 6, 2010, from http://www.va.gov.ezproxy1.lib.asu.edu/oaa

Dolde, K. (2007). Pioneering work in wound care/gastroenterology. *News—Line for Nursing, 8*(40), 4–7.

Downs, F. S. (1991). Informing the media. *Nursing Outlook, 40,* 195.

Eddy, L. L. (2007). Evaluation research as academic scholarship. *Nursing Education Perspectives, 28*(2), 77–81.

Ede, A., & Cormack, L. B. (2004). *A history of science in society: From philosophy to utility.* Orchard Park, NY: Broadview Press/Addison-Wesley. Fagin, C. (2000). *Essays on nursing leadership.* New York: Springer.

Federwisch, A. (2007). Bright ideas: RNs creating a culture of change. *Nurse Week, 8*(12), 10–11. Fineout-Overholt, E., Melnyk, B. M., & Schultz, A. (2005). Transforming health care from the inside out: Advancing evidence based practice in the 21st century. *Journal of Professional Nursing, 21,* 335–344.

Gibbons, J., Limoges, C., Nowotny, H., Schwartzman, S., Scot, P., & Trow, M. (1994). *The new production of knowledge: The dynamics of science and research in contemporary societies.* Thousand Oaks, CA: Sage.

Grove, G. (1962). *Beethoven and his nine symphonies.* New York: Dover.

Higgins, P. A., & Moore, M. M. (2000). Levels of theoretical thinking in nursing. *Nursing Outlook, 48,* 179–183.

Horgan, J. (1996). *The end of science.* New York: Addison-Wesley.

Ingraham, C. (1998). *Architecture and the burdens of linearity.* New Haven, NJ: Yale University Press.

Johns, C. (2004). *Becoming a reflective practitioner* (2nd ed.). Malden, MA: Blackwell.

Keller, J. (2007). Yo-Yo Ma's edge effect. *Chronicle of Higher Education, 23,* B10–B13.

Kuhn, T. S. (1996). *The structure of scientific revolutions* (3rd ed.). Chicago: University of Chicago Press. (Original work published 1962)

Latour, B. (1999). *Pandora's hope: Essays on the reality of science studies.* Cambridge, MA: Harvard University Press.

Latour, B., & Woolgar, S. (1986). *Laboratory life: The construction of scientific facts.* Princeton, NJ: Princeton University Press.

Lenoir, T. (1997). *Instituting science: The cultural production of scientific disciplines.* Stanford, CA: Stanford University Press.

Long, K. (2004). Preparing nurses for the 21st century: Re-envisioning nursing education and practice. *Journal of Professional Nursing, 20*(2), 82–88.

Longino, H. E. (2002). *The fate of knowledge.* Princeton, NJ: Princeton University Press.

Lum, C. (2002). *Scientific thinking in speech and language therapy.* Mahwah, NJ: Lawrence Erlbaum.

Lynaugh, J. E., & Fagin, C. M. (2000). Nursing comes of age. In C. M. Fagin (Ed.), *Essays on nursing leadership* (pp. 35–53). New York: Springer.

Mangan, K. (2007). Looming shortages of doctors and nurses are intertwined, report says. In K. Mangan (Ed.). *The chronicle of higher education, today's news.* Retrieved December 6, 2010, from http://chronicle.com.ezproxy1.lib.asu.edu/daily/2007/07/2007070902n.html

Marrs, J., & Lowry, L. W. (2006). Nursing theory and practice: Connecting the dots. *Nursing Science Quarterly, 19*(2), 116–119.

Meleis, A. I., & Im, E. (1999). Transcending marginalization in knowledge development. *Nursing Inquiry, 6,* 94–102.

Montgomery, K. (2006). *How doctors think: Clinical judgment and the practice of medicine.* New York: Oxford University Press.

Neill, J. (2005). Recognizing patterns in the lives of women with multiple sclerosis. In C. Picard & D. Jones (Eds.), *Giving voice to what we know* (pp. 153–168). Boston: Jones and Bartlett.

Nelson, S., & Gordon, S. (Eds.). (2006). *The complexities of care: Nursing reconsidered.* Ithaca, NY: Cornell University Press.

Palmer, A. M., Burns, S., & Bulman, C. (1994). *Reflective practice in nursing: The growth of the professional practitioner.* Boston: Blackwell.

Peden-McAlpine, C., Tomlinson, P. S., Forneris, S. G., Genck, G., & Meiers, S. J. (2005). Evaluation of a reflective practice intervention to enhance family care. *Journal of Advanced Nursing, 49,* 494–501.

Peirce, C. S., Harshorne, C., & Weiss, P. (Eds.). (1934). *Charles Sanders Peirce: Collected papers.* Cambridge, MA: Harvard University Press.

Pesut, D. J., & Herman, J. (1999). *Clinical reasoning: The art & science of critical & creative thinking.* Albany, NY: Delmar.

Pickering, A. (1995). *The mangle of practice: Time, agency and science.* Chicago: University of Chicago Press.

Purkis, M. E., & Bjornsdottir, K. (2006). Intelligent nursing: Accounting for knowledge as action *in* practice. *Nursing Philosophy, 7,* 247–256.

Ratner, T. (2007). A unique type of talk therapy. *NurseWeek: Mountain West Edition, 8,* 13.

Rawnsley, M. M. (2000). Response to Leddy's "Toward a complementary perspective on world-views." *Nursing Science Quarterly, 13,* 230–233.

Reed, P. G. (1995). A treatise on nursing knowledge development for the 21st century: Beyond postmodernism. *Advances in Nursing Science, 17*(3), 70–84.

Reed, P. G. (2001, October). *An emancipatory model for knowledge development in nursing.* Paper presented at the Knowledge Impact Conference, Boston College School of Nursing, Boston.

Reed, P. G. (2006a). The practice turn in nursing epistemology. *Nursing Science Quarterly, 19*(1), 36–38.

Reed, P. G. (2006b). Neomodernism and evidence-based nursing: Implications for the production of nursing knowledge. *Nursing Outlook, 54*(1), 36–38.

Roberts, A. R., & Yeager, K. (2004). Systematic review of evidenced-based studies and practice-based research: How to search for, develop, and use them. In A. R. Roberts & K. Yeager (Eds.), *Evidence-based practice manual* (pp. 3–14). New York: Oxford University Press.

Rolfe, G. (1998). *Expanding nursing knowledge: Understanding and researching your own practice*. Woburn, MA: Butterworth-Heinemann.

Rolfe, G. (2006). Nursing praxis and the science of the unique. *Nursing Science Quarterly, 19*(1), 39–43.

Salas, A. S. (2005). Toward a North–South dialogue: Revisiting nursing theory (from the South). *Advances in Nursing Science, 28*(1), 17–24.

Schön, D. A. (1983). *The reflective practitioner: How professionals think in action*. New York: Basic Books.

Segal, E. T. (1985). Is nursing a profession? *Nursing, 85*(15), 40–43.

Seigfried, C. H. (1996). *Pragmatism and feminism: Reweaving the social fabric*. Chicago: University of Chicago Press.

Serres, M. (1995) *Conversations on science, culture, and time: Michel Serres with Bruno Latour* (R. Lapidus, Trans.). Ann Arbor: University of Michigan Press.

Sturman, S. (2006). On black-boxing gender: Some social questions for Bruno Latour. *Social Epistemology, 20*, 181–184.

Thatchenkery, T., & Chowdhry, D. (2007). *Appreciative inquiry and knowledge management: A social constructionist perspective*. Northampton, MA: Edward Elgar.

Trierweiler, S. J., & Stricker, G. (1998). *The scientific practice of professional psychology*. New York: Plenum.

Tucker, D. J., Garvin, C., & Sarri, R. (1997). *Integrating knowledge and practice*. Westport, CT: Praeger.

U.S. Department of Health and Human Resources & Health Resources and Services Administration. (2007). *The registered nurse population: Findings from the 2004 national sample survey of registered nurses*. Retrieved December 6, 2010, from http://bhpr.hrsa.gov/healthworkforce/rnsurvey04/3.htm

Interlude V

Steps in Reformulating a Nursing Practice Concept: Empowerment as an Example

Nelma B. Crawford Shearer
Pamela G. Reed

oncepts are critical elements in building knowledge. This chapter is intended to help you find a concept that you might be interested in exploring further through your studies or graduate research. Sometimes a concept of interest may be used or defined in a way that is not quite right by your judgment, beliefs, and experiences. Rather than abandon a potentially rich concept, you may reformulate (modify) the concept to fit your perspectives. This reformulation involves not only a sound literature review but also reflecting on two important dimensions in your professional life: your nursing experiences and your philosophic views (worldviews) about human health and nursing practice.

There are many "not quite right" concepts in the literature that, with some reformulation according to your nursing perspective, may open a pathway to a new theory for nursing practice. The concept of empowerment presented in this chapter was my (NS) gateway to a theory about promoting the purposeful participation of homebound older women in their health and health care decisions. It emerged from experiences in practice, my Rogerian worldview, and ideas gleaned through concept analysis and clarification conducted in graduate coursework.

We invite you to read this chapter as an example of concept reformulation and then experiment with your own ideas about potential concepts related to practice for inquiry.

> I listened to the audio-tapes recorded for my research project while the nurses participating in the telephone intervention study talked and listened to the participants. Listening to the tapes has been an education in itself. While reviewing the tapes, it

Adapted by permission of Sage Publications, Inc. from Shearer, N. B. C., & Reed, P. G. (2004). Empowerment: Reformulation of a non-Rogerian concept. *Nursing Science Quarterly, 17*(3), pp. 253–259.

became apparent that one of the nurses making the telephone calls does not listen to the participant although I am sure she would strongly disagree with me. She is bent on getting the study participant to exercise and drink water. One participant in particular refers to listening to her body and states, "I know when something is wrong." The nurse responds by telling her she should instead talk with her doctor.

(Notes Recorded by a Rogerian Research Nurse, March 18, 2002)

The lack of knowledge and misuse of power in health care by the nurse in this audiotape not only reduced the patient's power to participate in the health process but also effectively diminished the nurse's own power as a facilitator of health care. This excerpt is an example of a practice experience that inspired the idea of reformulating the concept of empowerment so as to emphasize a participative, not paternalistic, approach to helping patients change their health patterns.

Reformulation involves a series of steps, beginning with the existing concept and concluding with the reformulated concept. It begins with a clarification about the author's philosophic views about nursing and human health, as they influence what ideas are used to modify the concept. Reformulation also includes a review of basic definitions of the concept, historical perspectives, and paradigmatic views from various disciplines that influence current thought on empowerment. A review of the research literature and a concept analysis may also be conducted early on in the reformulation. Next, the assumptions and principles of relevant nursing and nonnursing theories are considered. It is also an important step to critically address the nursing practice paradigms that may influence translation of the concept into action.

PHILOSOPHICAL RATIONALE FOR REFORMULATING

From a philosophy of science perspective, modifying existing concepts, ideas, or theories is an accepted practice in science. Philosophers support this as an approach to knowledge development. Nurse theoretician Whall (1980), drawing from philosopher of science Kaplan's (1964) ideas on the autonomy of inquiry, instructed scholars that concepts and theories are not owned by any one discipline and may be reformulated according to their own disciplinary perspective and purposes.

From a moral perspective, it may be wise to reformulate rather than *ignore* or continue using concepts and theories that are incongruent with a disciplinary perspective. As nurses, we believed in the benefits of a nursing perspective in health care and thought that the attitude conveyed by the nurse in the notes above conflicted with good nursing care. In this case, for example, reformulating the concept of empowerment was an opportunity to clarify and suggest new thinking about a fairly common approach to positively influence nurses' everyday interactions with patients.

After considering rationale for reformulating empowerment and determining it was an important phase in developing a theory of health empowerment (Shearer, 2007), several steps were followed. We describe each step briefly and then elaborate on our work as an example of the step. The general focus of each of these steps can be applied to modifying other concepts.

STEPS IN REFORMULATING A CONCEPT

STEP 1. CLARIFY YOUR PERSPECTIVE OF NURSING

Clarifying our theoretical perspective was useful in synthesizing a coherent and philosophically relevant reformulation of empowerment out of the wide variety of theories (nursing and nonnursing) about the concept. The reformulation was based on Rogerian nursing principles (Rogers, 1980, 1990, 1992) and the shift from positivist philosophy to philosophic views that supported a participative approach of helping patients change their health patterns.

Rogers (1980, 1990, 1992) defined nursing's focus as the study of human beings in mutual process with the environment. Rogers proposed three principles of homeodynamics, which outline her assumptions about the nature of the human–environment process as well as guide nursing practice. The principle of helicy describes the nature of human change as continuous, innovative, unpredictable, and reflective of the diversity of human and environment patterns. The principle of integrality proposes how this change occurs, that is through a continuous mutual process of human and environmental systems. The idea is that human beings and environment evolve in action together rather than as separated entities in reaction against each other. The principle of resonancy emphasizes the existence of patterns rather than parts that characterize human beings and their environment. Knowledge about these patterns are acquired through research and careful assessment and can then be used to facilitate health.

STEP 2. EXAMINE AND EVALUATE EXISTING DEFINITIONS AND DESCRIPTIONS OF THE CONCEPT

Dictionary definitions of empowerment are "(1) to give official authority or legal power to; (2) to enable; (3) to promote self-actualization or influence of" (*Merriam-Webster's Collegiate Dictionary*, 1993, p. 379). The prefix *em* in empowerment means "to cause to be," "to put into," "to provide with" (*Merriam-Webster's Collegiate Dictionary*, 1993, p. 379).

Empowerment is a ubiquitous concept not only in the health care literature but also across many social disciplines. In general, it connotes active participation in one's own health care. Furthermore, moral views and behaviors, personal integrity, and a sense of personal and social responsibility have been found to be qualities of empowerment (Kuokkanen, Leino-Kilpi, & Katajisto, 2002). Empowerment is generally associated with increased self-esteem and self-worth, inner confidence, and well-being (e.g., Gibson, 1991; Kieffer, 1984; Nyatanga & Dann, 2002).

Barrett, Caroselli, Smith, and Smith (1997) pointed out that the term's literal definition, to *put power into* an individual, reflects a mechanistic view of human beings in terms of the person passively receiving something from another. The definition also suggests an authoritative view of nursing, with the nurse as the primary one with the power and authority. Both of these views were evaluated as being incongruent with a nursing perspective, particularly given Rogers' (1980, 1990, 1992) descriptions of human beings and nursing practice.

STEP 3. REVIEW THE HISTORY OF THE CONCEPT

According to Minkler and Wallerstein (1997), the word *empowerment* first appeared in the literature during the 1950s, a time of social action organization in which the emphasis was on addressing power imbalances. Empowerment rooted in social action became more influential throughout the 1960s and 1970s within the contexts of civil rights, the women's movement, gay rights, the disability rights movement, and other community-based action. During the 1980s, in the psychology literature, empowerment was viewed as a participatory process through which individuals take control over their lives and environment (Rappaport, 1984). It was not until the 1990s, when health care providers' and consumers' focus turned to health promotion that the concept appeared on a regular basis in the nursing and health education literature.

In the context of health education, empowerment has been viewed as a process and an outcome; as a process, empowerment involves relationships and the transfer of the power base from one group to another, with the outcome of "liberation, emancipation, energy and sharing power" (Leyshon, 2002, p. 467). Empowerment can be understood from various broad perspectives. The social and the contextual developmental comprise two major perspectives.

STEP 4. REVIEW CURRENT PERSPECTIVES, ASSUMPTIONS, AND THEORIES RELATED TO THE CONCEPT

Given nursing's basic assumptions about the importance of human potential and development, connectedness, and the social context in health and well-being, both the social and developmental paradigms offer ideas that are useful in reformulating the concept of empowerment.

Social Paradigms

As a social process, empowerment is linked with external social forces that act on the individual and affect one's sense of control and feelings of power. For example, social support as an external feedback mechanism has been studied as a process that can provide needed reinforcement, resources, assistance, and motivation (Ellis-Stoll & Popkess-Vawter, 1998) and enable the individual (Hawks, 1992). Other external social forces have been studied from the perspective of emancipation from oppression. Several authors have suggested that promoting empowerment could be accomplished through addressing political (Gutierrez, 1995; Labonte, 1994), environmental (Ryles, 1999), and social constraints (Fulton, 1997). Two theories addressing these constraints are critical social theory and feminist theory, which offer perspectives about power applicable in nursing.

Critical social theory evolved from Marxism during the postmodern era and from the revolutionary thinking of Paulo Freire (1968/1981) in Brazil. Freire's basic assumption is that human being's "ontological vocation is to be a Subject who acts upon and transforms one's world" (Richard Shaull, as cited in Freire, 1968/1981, p. 12). The goals of critical social theory are to make people aware of the social constraints under which they may be consciously or unconsciously living, free people's thinking, and establish unconstrained communication.

Feminist thought of the 1960s extended the suffragists' cause of the late 19th through early 20th century to address the educational, occupational, professional, and role-related constraints experienced by women. Although diverse views on feminism exist, a unifying theme is the elimination of patriarchal social constraints and the oppression of women (Kirkley, 2000). Feminist theory acknowledges basic human potential in all human beings and incorporates interactions and life experiences that contribute to human transformation; this transformation of oppressive situations facilitates empowerment (Kane & Thomas, 2000). Empowerment from a feminist perspective draws from the ideology of equality by emphasizing the choices and freedom of women (Caroselli, 1995).

More recently, *postmodern feminism* has introduced a multicultural and global focus in which differences in race, class, national origin, and gender are regarded as relevant in the discourse on constraints on women's freedom and well-being (Tong, 2001). Postcolonial feminist theory has shifted away from the earlier emphasis on achieving a unified notion of women toward developing an appreciation of differences while holding a collective goal of equal opportunity. There is less of a stance of victimization and a more creative, proactive approach to one's social environment that develops the human potential of all (Ramphele, 1997).

Developmental Paradigm

Empowerment may also be understood in reference to the lifespan developmental perspective that emerged in the late 1970s (Lerner, 1997). Lifespan development is an orientation to the study of human beings as continuously innovative, embedded in a dynamic environment, and possessing inherent potential. The lifespan developmental perspective emphasizes both *systematic* patterns of change, such as biologically based influences, and *nonnormative* patterns of change across the lifespan, such as life events that cannot be predicted by time and do not occur for everyone. Development is no longer viewed as a linear process as it was until the late 20th century. Rather, developmental change is now understood to derive unpredictably from mutual influences between person and environmental contexts. Person–environment processes, including those involving human relationships, are central to developmental progress and well-being.

Treatment approaches from a lifespan view focus on maximizing client strengths and minimizing weaknesses (Baltes, Lindenberger, & Staudinger, 1998) rather than on predetermined interventions designed to change client behaviors. The client is regarded as possessing a repertoire of developmentally based abilities that can be educed through the nurse–client relationship to address health care needs. From this perspective, the client is a resource and active partner in health care. Nursing care is directed less toward changing the client and more toward optimizing human potential.

Related Nursing Theories

Several theoretical frameworks support the Rogerian postulate that human beings desire to participate knowingly in change and in their patterning. This idea has a central place in Barrett et al.'s (1997) power enhancement, Newman's (1997) expanding consciousness, and Reed's (1997) participatory nursing process. Synthesis of ideas from these frameworks supports a reformulation of the concept of empowerment.

BARRETT. Barrett's (1990) theory of *power as knowing participation in change* is similar to, but still qualitatively different from, typical views of empowerment. Barrett's underlying assumption about participation in ongoing change is a unique perspective. Basic to Barrett's (1990, 1994) theory of power is the assumption of ongoing change and the client's awareness of and belief in one's ability to fully participate in the changes involved in health and health care. The partnership between client and nurse facilitates the client's participation in health care. During the health-seeking event, the participatory nurse–client relationship evolves. The nurse uses various methods that enhance the client's knowing participation in change. One such approach centers on finding out what is happening with the client, directing attention away from the nurse as the initiator of nursing care and toward a participatory relationship in which both the nurse and client facilitate the change process. The nursing goal is "power enhancement through changing the environment" (Barrett et al., 1997, p. 34).

NEWMAN. Newman's (1997) theory of health as expanding consciousness proposes a mutual process between client and nurse by which meaning and understanding of the client's health patterns are recognized and insight is gained. The nurse does not attempt to control the interaction and change the client. Instead, the nurse facilitates pattern recognition and health choices faced by the client (Newman, 1990). This process of pattern recognition expands the client's developing insight and facilitates potential action.

REED. Reed (1997) described nursing as a "participatory process that transcends the boundary between patient and nurse" (p. 77). She defined nursing as an inherent process of well-being that functions within and among human systems. Reed explained that nursing, in its most basic meaning, is not an external process of 19th-century invention; rather it is a resource that has existed among human beings ever since the beginning of human history. Empowerment is an expression and indicator of this inherent nursing process. From this participatory perspective, empowerment is inherent in the nurse–client system rather than located in either the nurse or client alone. The process promotes well-being through the power inherent in this integrality of client and nurse.

STEP 5. REVIEW USES OF THE CONCEPT FROM THE PERSPECTIVES OF NURSING PRACTICE PARADIGMS

Parse (1987, 1992) identified two nursing paradigms, *totality* and *simultaneity*, that can guide thinking about nursing practice concepts. A Rogerian view of empowerment is congruent with the simultaneity paradigm of nursing practice.

Totality

According to the totality paradigm, humans are biopsychosocial-spiritual beings interacting with and in response to the internal and external environment (Parse, 1992). Human change is considered predictable, controllable, and occurring primarily in response to environmental stimuli. Health is viewed as achieving equilibrium in physical, mental, social, and spiritual dimensions. Within this paradigm, the nurse knows what is best for the client and uses the nurse–client relationship to influence change in the desired direction. Empowerment is accomplished through the efforts of the nurse as data collector, assessor of the disease state, care planner, and change agent for the client. The nurse as the authority shares knowledge to empower the client to make informed choices that are appropriate and in compliance with the care plan.

Simultaneity

Within the simultaneity paradigm (Parse, 1992), human beings are recognized through pattern rather than through parts that can be independently manipulated, changed, and studied. Change is creative and innovative and occurs as part of the person–environment process. Health involves the client's purposeful participation in developing self-awareness and choosing health patterns. Clients exercise their power by participating in their health care and health care decisions. The nurse's approach is to inspire, not dictate this process; to be facilitative, not authoritative.

Uses of the Concept

It is not uncommon for health care providers to think that they can empower their clients and in so doing expect clients will comply with the health plan (e.g., Hawks, 1992; Holmes & Saleebey, 1993). Empowerment is often implicitly, if not explicitly, linked to the concept of compliance in practice. The concept neither appeals to the informed consumer nor reflects contemporary nursing philosophy of science. Clinical practice and anecdotal experiences consistently indicate that clients do not always follow through with the nurse's prescribed plan of care (Hess, 1996). The nurse, thinking that the client has been amply empowered, may be puzzled as to why the person does not *comply* with the health care plan.

Confounding empowerment and compliance is insidious and prevails even in very recent literature appearing to advance understandings of empowerment beyond authoritarian assumptions, for example, "non-compliance demonstrated the patient's need to exercise their empowerment" (Nyatanga & Dann, 2002, p. 238), as though noncompliance really exists in patients and is linked to empowerment. The authors go on to explain that the nursing discipline should cease using the term *patients*, come around to the true philosophy of empowerment, and relinquish the discipline's authoritarian approach. However, the problem is not so much the lack of the correct understanding of empowerment as it is the nurse's practice paradigm (perspective) that influences applications of empowerment.

EMPOWERMENT REFORMULATED

Rogers did not specifically address empowerment in publications on her science of unitary human beings. Nonetheless, her theoretical views were helpful in synthesizing ideas from social and developmental theories. From Rogers (1992), it is understood that there is an emphasis on participating knowingly in the process of change rather than on submission and lack of power, control, or choice. Attention to external agents of power are inconsistent with these assumptions. The nurse is not one who empowers but rather one who facilitates empowerment in clients, with actions deriving from an understanding of the client's relational nature, relevant social context, and developmental potential.

This new view of empowerment is based on four assumptions derived from Rogerian theory and related theories: (a) Empowerment is neither a resource that is external to the person nor bestowed by others, power is inherent and ongoing (Labonte, 1989); (b) empowerment is a relational process, expressive of the mutuality of person and environment; (c) empowerment is an ongoing process of change that is continuously innovative; and (d) empowerment is expressive of a human health pattern of well-being and can be assessed and enhanced through nursing knowledge, including practice and science-based inquiry.

Empowerment as reformulated, then, is defined as *a health patterning of well-being in which the client optimizes the ability to transform self through the relational process of nursing.* It may involve identifying and transcending sources of oppression that constrain human potential and limit self-understanding of personal resources. The Rogerian ideas of Barrett et al.'s (1997) power enhancement, Newman's (1997) expanding consciousness and Reed's (1997) participatory process of well-being together provide for a reformulated view of empowerment—one that extends the possibilities of change for all participants (Cowling, 2001) as a dynamic human health process. Empowerment can then be understood as a complex and participatory process of changing oneself and one's environment, recognizing patterns, and engaging inner resources for well-being. It is a process greater than any one theory can represent. It is a process that is central to a unitary perspective of human beings (Cowling, 2001).

A CASE STUDY

The following story illustrates the experience of empowerment and offers an example of the mutual process of power that is inherent in the nurse–client system. Susan, a community health nurse, focuses on patterning the environment with Ida to promote Ida's sense of power to participate in health care and health care decisions. In talking with Ida, Susan focuses on Ida's strengths, facilitates a supportive relational process, and provides empowering education that promotes Ida's health.

Several years ago, Susan met Ida during a home visit. Ida was in her late 70s, diagnosed with chronic obstructive pulmonary disease (COPD), osteoporosis, and heart failure. She was on many medications, including nebulizer treatments, inhalers, continuous oxygen, and pills. Ida had been in the hospital frequently for COPD exacerbations. She told Susan that she did not like going to the hospital: "They didn't do much for me other than increasing my breathing treatments and giving me IV steroids," and "I can do that at home."

Ida lived with her son, daughter-in-law, and their two children. She had an upstairs bedroom and stayed there except for meals, which she would take down in the kitchen if her breathing would allow it. She said the family did not provide her with much support, and often she would go for days without anyone coming in to say "hi." Ida was lonely. She filled her time with crafts including crocheting and making items with beads plus she liked to read and watch video movies. She told Susan she did not know where a couple of her children were and she had a daughter in prison for armed robbery. She communicated with this daughter through letters and they provided each other with support.

When Susan first met Ida, Ida was a little skeptical. She told Susan later that she did not know what a nurse would be able to do for her and that she had been used to taking care of herself and her own health. They discussed Ida's health, and Susan provided her with information on ways that she could take care of herself so she would not have frequent exacerbations and end up in the hospital. They talked about daily weighing and she got permission from the physician to take extra Lasix if her weight increased. Ida and Susan talked about Ida's frequent breathing crises and the importance of catching things early. They also talked about listening to her body and being in tune with her breathing pattern. Ida started being more *in tune* with her body and being aware of when she needed to call the physician for an antibiotic or an increase in Prednisone to prevent further complications.

Ida developed moon face and was also having neck pain from the damage that had been caused by taking Prednisone. She wanted to stop taking it, but whenever she asked the physician he said, "No." Ida and Susan talked about it, and Susan supported her in her efforts. They talked about the risks (and the benefits) of being off Prednisone, and Ida made her decision. She weaned herself off very gradually and was successful in staying off except when she would get a bad cold or infection.

Ida began to feel so good that she began to verbalize that perhaps she could get out of her children's hair and get her own place. Ida and Susan talked about her options, including the possibility of moving into a group home or an assisted living arrangement. Unfortunately, due to Ida's limited income, she was unable to move from her children's home, but she decided that she could get out of the house during the day to participate in group activities. Susan and Ida visited two senior centers and determined together which one had programs that fit Ida's interests.

Susan no longer has Ida as a client. Ida moved out of state and lives with her daughter. Susan shared that she learned a great deal from Ida, especially about the importance of a person actively participating in the ongoing changes in their health and the ever-present potential for well-being.

> Ida told me she appreciated that I encouraged her to participate in the decisions regarding her own life and health. But really what happened was that Ida became aware of her ability to actively participate in making health decisions. She just needed to be educated on a better way of handling things and then needed the support to do it. She taught me what it is like to live with chronic illness and yet look forward to every day.

Thus, Ida was empowered by this participatory mutual process in which the nurse nurtured Ida's ability to recognize her pattern of well-being and her natural resources for healing self. In addition, the nurse was empowered by facilitating the mutual process of innovative change for the client.

SUMMARY

Rogerian science was used to synthesize a new view of empowerment out of social and developmental perspectives. The reformulation is consistent with nursing assumptions about patterns of human health and change. It is also congruent with the simultaneity paradigm of nursing practice. Reformulation of the concept involved a shift in focus from empowerment for clients to the relational process of empowerment within and among human systems, nurse and client alike.

This shift in thinking that occurred at a concept level has yet to be fully realized in nursing practice. The proposed view alters the traditional paternalistic focus in health care systems that minimizes the individual's identity, choice, and participation in health, and in so doing, minimizes the role of nursing overall. As Kane and Thomas (2000) have suggested, a disempowered profession cannot empower clients.

Empowerment represents a dynamic human health process, one of many that nursing seeks to understand for the betterment of society. By enacting a worldview that acknowledges empowerment as a nursing process inherent in and among human beings, nurses relinquish an authoritarian nursing process external to the person. Nurses and clients may work together more equally and effectively to promote health and well-being and thereby, move nursing from the practice to the praxis of empowerment.

QUESTIONS FOR REFLECTION

1. What concept interests you as related to your nursing practice? Think about how you might decide on a concept related to practice.
2. How would you define your concept according to your knowledge and views about human health and nursing practice?

REFERENCES

Baltes, P. B., Lindenberger, U., & Staudinger, U. M. (1998). Life-span theory in developmental psychology. In R. Lerner (Ed.), *Theoretical models of human development* (pp. 1029–1143). New York: John Wiley.

Barrett, E. A. M. (1990). Health patterning with clients in a private practice environment. In E. A. M. Barrett (Ed.), *Visions of Rogers' science-based nursing* (pp. 105–115). New York: National League for Nursing.

Barrett, E. A. M. (1994). Rogerian scientists, artists, revolutionaries. In M. Madrid & E. A. M. Barrett (Eds.), *Rogers' scientific art of nursing practice* (pp. 61–87). New York: National League for Nursing.

Barrett, E. A. M., Caroselli, C., Smith, A. S., & Smith, D. W. (1997). Power as knowing participation in change: Theoretical, practice, and methodological issues, insights, and ideas. In M. Madrid (Ed.), *Patterns of Rogerian knowing* (pp. 31–46). New York: National League for Nursing.

Caroselli, C. (1995). Power and feminism: A nursing science perspective. *Nursing Science Quarterly, 8,* 115–119.

Cowling, W. R. (2001). Unitary appreciative inquiry. *Advances in Nursing Science, 23*(4), 32–48.

Ellis-Stoll, C., & Popkess-Vawter, S. (1998). A concept analysis on the process of empowerment. *Advances in Nursing Science, 21*(2), 62–68.

Freire, P. (1981). *Pedagogy of the oppressed* (M. B. Ramos, Trans.). New York: Continuum. (Original work published 1968)

Fulton, Y. (1997). Nurses' views on empowerment: A critical social theory perspective. *Journal of Advanced Nursing, 26,* 529–536.

Gibson, C. H. (1991). A concept analysis of empowerment. *Journal of Advanced Nursing, 16,* 344–561.

Gutierrez, L. (1995). Understanding the empowerment process: Does consciousness make a difference? *Social Work Research, 19,* 229–237.

Hawks, J. (1992). Empowerment in nursing education: Concept analysis and application to philosophy, learning and instruction. *Journal of Advanced Nursing, 17,* 609–618.

Hess, J. (1996). The ethics of compliance: A dialectic. *Advances in Nursing Science, 19*(1), 18–27.

Holmes, G., & Saleebey, D. (1993). Empowerment, the medical model, and the politics of clienthood. *Journal of Progressive Human Services, 4*(1), 61–78.

Kane, D., & Thomas, B. (2000). Nursing and the "F" word. *Nursing Forum, 35*(2), 17–24.

Kaplan, A. (1964). *The conduct of inquiry.* New York: Thomas Y. Crowell.

Kieffer, C. (1984). Citizen empowerment: A developmental perspective. *Prevention in Human Services, 3,* 9–36.

Kirkley, D. (2000). Is motherhood good for women? A feminist exploration. *Journal of Obstetrics, Gynecologic and Neonatal Nursing, 29,* 459–464.

Kuokkanen, L., Leino-Kilpi, H., & Katajisto, J. (2002). Do nurses feel empowered? Nurses' assessment of their own qualities and performance with regard to nurse empowerment. *Journal of Professional Nursing, 18,* 328–335.

Labonte, R. (1989). Community and professional empowerment. *Canadian Nurse, 85*(3), 23–28.

Labonte, R. (1994). Health promotion and empowerment: Reflections on professional practice. *Health Education Quarterly, 21,* 253–268.

Lerner, R. (1997). *Concepts and theories of human development* (2nd ed.). Mahwah, NJ: Lawrence Erlbaum.

Leyshon, S. (2002). Empowering practitioners: An unrealistic expectation of nurse education? *Journal of Advanced Nursing, 40,* 466–474.

Minkler, M., & Wallerstein, N. (1997). Improving health through community organization and community building. In K. Glanz, F. Lewis, & B. Rimer (Eds.), *Health behavior and health education: Theory, research, and practice* (2nd ed., pp. 241–269). San Francisco: Jossey-Bass.

Merriam-Webster's collegiate dictionary. (10th ed.). (1993). Springfield, MA: Merriam-Webster.

Newman, M. (1990). Shifting to higher consciousness. In M. Parker (Ed.), *Nursing theories in practice* (pp. 129–139). New York: National League for Nursing.

Newman, M. (1997). Evolution of the theory of health as expanding consciousness. *Nursing Science Quarterly, 10,* 22–25.

Nyatanga, L., & Dann, K. L. (2002). Empowerment in nursing: The role of philosophical and psychological factors. *Nursing Philosophy, 3,* 234–239.

Parse, R. R. (1987). Paradigms and theories. In R. R. Parse (Ed.), *Nursing science: Major paradigms, theories, and critiques* (pp. 1–11). Philadelphia: Saunders.

Parse, R. R. (1992). Human becoming: Parse's theory of nursing. *Nursing Science Quarterly, 5,* 35–42.

Ramphele, M. (1997). Whither feminism? In J. Scott, C. Kaplan, & D. Keates (Eds.), *Transitions, environments, translations* (pp. 334–338). New York: Routledge.

Rappaport, J. (1984). Studies in empowerment: Introduction to the issue. *Prevention in Human Services, 3,* 1–7.

Reed, P. G. (1997). Nursing: The ontology of the discipline. *Nursing Science Quarterly, 10,* 76–79.

Rogers, M. E. (1980). A science of unitary man. In J. P. Riehl & C. Roy (Eds.), *Conceptual models for nursing practice* (2nd ed., pp. 329–337). New York: Appleton-Century-Crofts.

Rogers, M. E. (1990). Nursing: Science of unitary, irreducible, human beings: Update 1990. In E. A. M. Barrett (Ed.), *Visions of Rogers' science-based nursing* (pp. 5–11). New York: National League for Nursing.

Rogers, M. E. (1992). Nursing science and space age. *Nursing Science Quarterly, 5,* 27–34.

Ryles, S. (1999). A concept analysis of empowerment: Its relationship to mental health nursing. *Journal of Advanced Nursing, 29,* 600–607.

Shearer, N. B. C. (2007). Toward a nursing theory of health empowerment in homebound older women. *Journal of Gerontological Nursing, 33*(12), 38–45.

Tong, R. (2001). A millennial feminist vision. In J. P. Sterba (Ed.), *Controversies in feminism* (pp. 173–195). Lanham, MD: Rowman & Littlefield.

Whall, A. (1980). Congruence between existing theories of family functioning and nursing theories. *Advances in Nursing Science, 3*(1), 59–67.

12

The Practice Turn in Nursing Epistemology

Pamela G. Reed

This chapter brings the book to an end by revisiting an idea that initiated this book; that is, the idea that nursing knowledge development is integral with nursing practice, wherever it occurs as a process of facilitating human health and well-being. Nursing practice typically has been viewed as a *context for applying* knowledge or theory but not as a *process of developing* knowledge. With the shift in the educational philosophy toward increasing the numbers of graduate-level nurses, nursing has an opportunity to extend knowledge-production resources into nursing practice. For this to happen, though, there needs to be an accompanying shift in our philosophy of knowledge development in nursing.

The *turn* in this chapter refers to a change in focus—one that expands the traditional approach to linking theory and practice in *theory-guided practice* to include a focus on *practice-based theory development*. With this philosophic perspective about knowledge (i.e., epistemology), nurses may engage in theory development that is more context relevant and *patient centered*. As you read, I invite you to reflect on these ideas in reference to your own nursing practice.

Nursing is a fascinating discipline. Nurses have the honor and expertise to participate closely in human healing processes of individuals, families, and communities. Yet, because the practitioner's expertise in healing is not fully understood, some account for it by relying on concepts (like intuition, tacit knowing, and gut feelings) that render nursing knowledge more mystical than professional. Admittedly, there are elements of mystery in nurses' patterns of knowing, just as there is mystery that accompanies scientific knowledge in general (e.g., Adam, 2009; Raymo, 2006). However, contrary to philosophers of science Reichenbach and Popper, the *context of discovery* is not primarily mystical territory (Lamb & Easton, 1984). I think it is both possible and beneficial to pursue fuller explanations of how nursing knowledge is produced in the context of practice. Furthermore, trends in practice regarding evidence-based nursing, an intensified interest in advanced practice degrees,

Adapted with permission of Sage Publications, Inc. from Reed, P. G. (2006). The practice turn in nursing epistemology. *Nursing Science Quarterly, 19*(1), pp. 36–38.

and the rise of the Doctor of Nursing Practice degree degree all necessitate inquiry into nursing's epistemological infrastructure. So in this chapter, I have proposed rationale and a perspective for thinking anew about knowledge production in nursing practice.

For too long, nurses and other practicing professionals have more or less accepted the idea of a theory–practice gap and viewed science as distinct from a discipline's art or practice. The researcher has been portrayed as the *producer* who hands down scientific knowledge to the clinician as the *applier* of knowledge, sometimes *supplier* of ideas or researchable problems, maybe even *tester* of knowledge, but rarely *producer* of knowledge and theory. This traditional model of nursing knowledge production may not only misrepresent and constrain the knowledge potential in nursing but also marginalize the practitioner and distance patients from the process of knowledge development. There is a need for philosophical inquiry into beliefs and values about the "truest" or best source of nursing knowledge. In addition, there is a need for empirical inquiry into whether and how nurses produce knowledge through their practice. The results are likely to extend the science of nursing practice well beyond descriptions of intuition and gut feelings and even beyond current descriptions of critical thinking and clinical reasoning.

Granted, knowledge from nursing and other sciences developed outside of nursing practice can be useful for application, perhaps with needed translation or reformulation. However, to the extent that nurses strive to facilitate patients' resources and participation in care and healing processes, it seems logical to include if not emphasize (over the researcher-centered model) a nurse–patient practice-centered model in developing scientific knowledge. For example, knowledge generated through practice can more effectively address the thorny epistemologic problem of "who can speak for others" (Alcoff, 1995) by enabling the nurse to speak not *for* the patient but *with* the patient.

Precursors to this *practice turn*—so called by Rouse (2002)—in epistemology were evident in nursing more than a half-century ago. In addition, during the last decade, scholars within and outside of nursing increasingly acknowledged the role of human practices in knowledge production and critiqued orthodox epistemology with its one path to scientific knowledge.

NURSING

Mining for ideas about nursing knowledge in the conceptual models and theorists' publications turned up several statements where scholars had specifically described practitioners as knowledge producers. More than 50 years ago, Peplau (1952, 1992) presented her *cycle of inquiry* whereby the practitioner transformed practice knowledge into nursing knowledge. Peplau (1952, 1992) explained that the practicing nurse peels out theoretical explanations and formulates hypotheses, which are then validated and tested in the context of the nurse–patient relationship (Reed, 1996). Ellis (1969) conceptualized the *practitioner as theorist* and plainly stated that the practitioner was "not simply a user of given theory but a developer, tester, and expander of theory" (p. 1438). Paterson and Zderad (1976) outlined five phases in nursology, the phenomenological study of nursing practice. Researcher and practitioner roles were integrated and nurse–patient interactions produced theoretical *conceptions* derived from the local situation that held meaning across multiple situations. Roy (Roy & Obloy, 1978) described the practitioner as building knowledge through practice and, in fact, defined this as the process of nursing science. Diers' (1995) exemplary work on clinical scholarship paved a way for clinicians to raise their clinical observations and stories to the "level of theory" (p. 27). The next century brought an increasing number of nursing publications focused on nursing praxis as the *inseparability of theory/practice* (e.g., Connor, 2004; Doane & Varcoe, 2005; Rolfe, 1996, 2000).

SCIENCE STUDIES

Outside of nursing, sociology and culture scholars from the field of science studies (see Hess, 1997, for an overview) and the writings by historians and philosophers of science indirectly provide vigorous support for promoting nursing practice as integral to nursing knowledge and theory production. For example, Gibbons et al. (1994) proposed the now popular Mode 2 form of knowledge production that supplements traditional Mode 1 research approaches. Within the Mode 2 approach, knowledge evolves close to the *context of application* and, in fact, knowledge is legitimized by its use. Pickstone (2000) theorized that ways of knowing are linked to one's work and ways of making things. The practice-centered philosophy of Shusterman (1997) suggests that the embodied experiences of practicing and receiving nursing care, and then reflecting on these events, comprise a process that generates new knowledge. In addition, Baird's (2004) philosophic inquiry into technology established important links between the intelligent use of instruments in practice and scientific knowledge. So a nurse's interface with technology in patient care provides another opportunity for knowledge production in the context of practice.

In addition, historians have clarified that science itself is a practice and one that is much messier than what is portrayed in traditional descriptions of research. For example, Pickering (1995) described science as a *mangle* of social, technical, conceptual, political, and personal practices.

It is uncertain whether practicing nurses will embrace the practice turn in epistemology. Nevertheless, findings from Abbott's (1988) research into professions indicate that practitioners and the profession as a whole would benefit from theory-based knowledge production in practice. Based on his study of professions, Abbott concluded that *abstract thinking* was a dominant factor in determining whether professions had full jurisdiction over their practice. In his 1988 book, Abbott identified nursing as an exemplar of a profession with limited jurisdiction, implying that nursing lacked sufficient activity of abstract thinking in practice. Is this still so? Or do nurses peel out concepts and theories from their interactions with patients to produce practice knowledge? A study by Larsen, Adamsen, Bjerregaard, and Madsen

(2002) found that clinical nurses identified various sources of knowledge but denied using or producing theory in their practice.

TOWARD A MODEL OF KNOWLEDGE PRODUCTION

I suggest that knowledge production be conceptualized as integral with practice, patient centered, and theory based and that practicing nurses be viewed as eminently capable of integrating theoretical thinking with data from patient interactions to develop knowledge and theories relevant to patient care. Theorizing in practice is a creative process that can be studied, taught, and facilitated. To theorize is to think abstractly and make links between the empirical and conceptual. Practitioners who function as theory-based knowledge producers can help bring about the discipline's realization of full jurisdiction over nursing practice.

This model does not exclude the role of research in knowledge production. Partnerships between practitioners and researchers still hold, although research methods for practitioners need to be clarified or developed. The researcher typically practices science without direct experience in nursing practice and produces knowledge *of* nursing, employing systematic methods of scientific inquiry that emphasize the empirical patterns of knowing. The practitioner, however, practices science within the context of nursing care and produces knowledge *in* nursing by employing a wider array of patterns of knowing (aesthetic to technological and including empirical) to generate nursing theories.

Three basic assumptions underlie the model. These are as follows:

1. Nursing practice is a process of facilitating human processes of health and well-being.
2. The nursing practice setting is not only a place of knowledge application but also a context wherein nurse–patient encounters generate important data for building nursing knowledge.
3. Knowledge building involves abstract thought and generation or refinement of nursing theory, at some level of theory.

CAVEATS AND CONCLUSIONS

The characterizations of practitioner and researcher roles and other ideas that I have suggested in this chapter admittedly will benefit from more thought and dialogue and from research! The model begs for explanations about whether and how practicing nurses engage in roles of both practitioner and researcher to produce theory-based knowledge. Part of the answer lies in examining existing descriptions and theories about the various forms of human reasoning. Part of the answer will come from systematic study of practitioners and other caregivers in their daily work. And part of the answer resides in the philosophy, goals, and values nurses have about their science and practice.

There is increasing evidence in the literature of a convergence of thought occurring independently across scholars—a phenomenon Lamb and Easton (1984) called *multiple discoveries*—about nursing practice and knowledge. In other words, multiple people are expressing similar ideas about the significance of practice in the production of nursing knowledge and theory. I hope more nurses will consider the untapped role of practice in nursing knowledge production, will question traditional views of science that may subordinate clinicians' expert knowing, and will turn scholarly attention toward exploring what it means to know and who are the legitimate knowers in nursing. May more nurses join the multiple discoveries unfolding to advance the state of knowledge and theory production in nursing practice and to advance the status of the discipline and its capacity to facilitate human health and well-being.

QUESTIONS FOR REFLECTION

1. What role should nursing practice have in nursing theory and knowledge development?
2. What changes do practicing nurses need to support their knowledge-development activities in practice?
3. What changes need to occur in nursing education to facilitate development of practicing nurses as theory builders?
4. What new (and existing) research strategies and methods can be used to build knowledge and theory in practice?

REFERENCES

Abbott, A. (1988). *The system of professions*. Chicago: University of Chicago Press.

Adam, F. (2009). *The constant fire: Beyond the science vs. religion debate*. Berkeley: University of California Press.

Alcoff, L. M. (1995). The problem of speaking for others. In J. Roof & R. Wiegman (Eds.), *Who can speak? Authority and critical identity* (pp. 97–119). Chicago: University of Illinois Press.

Baird, D. (2004). *Thing knowledge: A philosophy of scientific instruments*. Los Angeles: University of California Press.

Connor, M. J. (2004). The practical discourse in philosophy and nursing: An exploration of linkages and shifts in the evolution of praxis. *Nursing Philosophy, 5*, 54–66.

Diers, D. (1995). Clinical scholarship. *Journal of Professional Nursing, 11*(1), 24–30.

Doane, G. H., & Varcoe, C. (2005). Toward compassionate action: Pragmatism and the inseparability of theory/practice. *Advances in Nursing Science, 28*(1), 81–90.

Ellis, R. (1969). The practitioner as theorist. *American Journal of Nursing, 68*, 1434–1438.

Gibbons, M., Limoges, C., Nowotny, H., Schwartzman, S., Scott, P., & Trow, M. (1994). *The new production of knowledge: The dynamics of science and research in contemporary societies*. Thousand Oaks, CA: Sage.

Hess, D. J. (1997). *Science studies: An advanced introduction*. New York: New York University Press.

Lamb, D., & Easton, S. M. (1984). *Multiple discovery: The pattern of scientific progress*. Trowbridge, UK: Avebury.

Larsen, K., Adamsen, L., Bjerregaard, L., & Madsen, J. K. (2002). There is no gap "per se" between theory and practice: Research knowledge and clinical knowledge are developed in different contexts and follow their own logic. *Nursing Outlook, 50,* 204–212.

Peplau, H. (1952). *Interpersonal relations in nursing*. New York: Putnam.

Peplau, H. (1992). Interpersonal relations: A theoretical framework for application in nursing practice. *Nursing Science Quarterly, 5,* 13–18.

Paterson, J., & Zderad, L. (1976). *Humanistic nursing*. New York: John Wiley.

Pickering, A. (1995). *The mangle of practice: Time, agency, and science*. Chicago: University of Chicago.

Pickstone, J. V. (2000). *Ways of knowing: A new history of science, technology and medicine*. Manchester, UK: Manchester University Press.

Raymo, C. (2006). *Walking zero: Discovering cosmic space and time along the Prime Meridian*. New York: Walker.

Reed, P. G. (1996). Transforming practice knowledge into nursing knowledge—A revisionist analysis of Peplau. *Image: Journal of Nursing Scholarship, 28*(1), 27–31.

Rolfe, G. (1996). *Closing the theory–practice gap: A new paradigm for nursing*. Oxford, UK: Butterworth-Heinemann.

Rolfe, G. (2000). *Nursing praxis and the reflexive practitioner: Collected papers 1993–1999*. London: NPI.

Rouse, J. (2002). *How scientific practices matter*. Chicago: University of Chicago Press.

Roy, C., & Obloy, M. (1978). The practitioner movement—Toward a science of nursing. *American Journal of Nursing, 10,* 1698–1702.

Shusterman, R. (1997). *Practicing philosophy: Pragmatism and the philosophical life*. New York: Routledge.

Index

Note: Page references followed by "*f*" and "*t*" denote figures and tables, respectively.